3-2-

ic

STUDENT·NURSE·SERIES

Essential Psychiatric Nursing

Robert G. Mitchell   RMN RGN RNT

Nurse Tutor, South Lothian College of
Nursing and Midwifery, Edinburgh

Foreword by
Professor Penny Prophit   BSN MSN DNSc PhD

Head of Department of Nursing Studies,
University of Edinburgh

Churchill Livingstone 🏛

EDINBURGH LONDON MELBOURNE AND NEW YORK 1986

CHURCHILL LIVINGSTONE
Medical Division of Longman Group Limited

Distributed in the United States of America by
Churchill Livingstone Inc., 1560 Broadway, New York,
N.Y. 10036, and by associated companies, branches
and representatives throughout the world.

First published 1986

ISBN 0-443-03246-7

British Library Cataloguing in Publication Data
Mitchell, Robert G.
    Essential psychiatric nursing. — (Student
    nurse series)
    1. Psychiatric nursing
    I. Title   II. Series
    610.73'68   RC440

Library of Congress Cataloging in Publication Data
Mitchell, Robert G.
    Essential psychiatric nursing.
    (Student nurse series)
    Includes bibliographies and index.
    1. Psychiatric nursing.   I. Title.   II. Series.
[DNLM: 1. Psychiatric Nursing. WY 160 M682e]
RC440.M58   1986   610.73'68   85–13220

Produced by Longman Singapore
Publishers (Pte) Ltd.
Printed in Singapore

Foreword

'Psychiatric nursing is about people ...'
... and this refreshing new book is unashamedly about psychiatric nursing and about people. It heralds an exciting and hopeful new era, with positive and inspiriting belief in behaviour as meaningful, purposeful and understandable if we would but try. Bob Mitchell is to be commended for recognizing a need, a compelling need in the literature of nursing. This work is a goldmine of information, and is written with an appreciation of the values which are inherent in patient-centred care through examples in practical situations, in simple language spiced with humour and sensitivity.

This book steps back from the usual posture which divides general and psychiatric nursing, recognizing that physically ill people have emotional selves and that psychological pain is frequently manifest in physical signs. The author confronts us with a view of persons as whole beings, and he is well qualified by experience and heart to write about psychiatric nursing. He is forthright in his eminently readable language style. He sets about describing in clinically-rich examples, issues and situations relevant to psychiatric nursing, in the awareness that trends and issues are more than the sum of their parts. He has recognized that it is necessary to go beyond itemizing and develop a larger vision of how issues meet and merge or find their resting place in conflict. As this book unfolds, it is the cumulative sense of the spirit and humanity of psychiatric nursing that forcefully impresses.

In a laudable fashion the author presents the values and concrete working through of the nursing process in the psychiatric context. He gives relevant examples of the concerns of psychiatric nursing in our modern times and the issues of increased incidence, whether speaking of anorexia as a self-destructive behaviour of our youth, involutional melancholia as a mid-life phenomenon, or dementia as the pervasive concern of aging. The reader learns that suicide is a kind of *cri de coeur* and gains from the incorporation of some of the latest research concerning the importance of reminscing in aging and as an intervention in dementia. One learns and enjoys while learning.

Respectful, realistic and sensitive to the vulnerability of the uninformed and those who are cared for by the uninformed, Bob Mitchell focuses on forces at work and the bringing together of nursing as a human science and art of caring for others.

Like Bob Mitchell, I strongly believe the directions of our future will be for good, and this book, by confronting us with the sense of history and with the awareness of the present as well as anticipation of the future, will help make it so.

I am sincerely grateful to him for this book, and we are all the beneficiaries of his dedicated labour of love.

Edinburgh 1986   Penny Prophit

Preface

This book is primarily aimed at nurses studying for the general register or roll. It is intended to provide a broad and uncontroversial introduction to psychiatric nursing and psychiatry.

While some readers will eagerly await their psychiatric module, perhaps sensing an affinity with the patients they will meet, others may be altogether uncertain about what they can expect. They may be conscious of being directed towards the speciality by the requirements of their training and may be unaware of having any great interest in the subject.

To them, my message is simple: go to it with enthusiasm! Psychiatric nursing should be both enlightening and enjoyable; let this book be the guide that helps make it so.

Hopefully, by reading it, learners will feel theoretically prepared both for their work on the wards and for the psychiatrically orientated questions in their examinations. But my ambitions go further. A second and sincere aim of this text is to demystify psychiatric nursing and to highlight the essentially human qualities of the psychiatrically disordered. Patients, after all, are people, and people can never say with any certainty that they will not one day be patients.

It was only after some deliberation that I chose to refer, on occasions, to my patients as schizophrenic, depressive and so on. This is because it has become fashionable to twist the English language in such a way as to avoid using what some people think are stigmatising and meaningless labels. They may have a point. However, by avoiding such words (which the nurse will most assuredly hear freely in her work), I fear I may succeed merely in baffling my readers, without in any way influencing for the better my philosophy of care. Therefore, I speak of schizophrenia, of confusion and of neurosis. I do so unashamedly and will feel regret only if, by the time they have finished my book, I have failed to convince my readers of the high regard and fond affection that I feel for the patients I have known, both past and present.

Edinburgh 1986   Robert G. Mitchell

Acknowledgements

During the writing of this book I sought, and was freely given, the expert advice of a number of colleagues and/or friends. In particular I acknowledge my debt to Ian Adams, Sheila Mackie, Harry Needham, Mac Rigg and Dave Stewart, although of course, responsibility for the text (including any errors) must be mine alone.

Janice White, the librarian, and Lyn McIntyre, who typed my script, responded with speed and good humour to my sometimes unreasonable requests. Ella Moir helped unsplit my infinitives and was unstinting in her advice, while as the deadline approached, Rena Rodger proved an invaluable Girl Friday.

I am deeply grateful to Professor Penny Prophit who agreed to write the foreword, and did so with great enthusiasm. Douglas Kirk brings his own inimitable style to the illustrations, while the staff of Churchill Livingstone proved invaluable mentors. I thank them all.

My own tenuous links with sanity were maintained by the patience and support of my wife, Anne, and the irrepressible antics of our three children. Nicola, Robert and Sam stayed quiet enough to let me write, but remained, I hope, sufficiently unfettered to avoid the trauma of a repressive childhood as described in the text. They made me laugh at times when things did not seem funny, and for that I thank them.

R.G.M.

Contents

ONE

The role of the nurse in psychiatry

1

Psychiatric nursing — past and present

Nowadays, people who exhibit disorders of thought, mood or emotion are usually described as being mentally ill, and care by doctors and nurses is considered appropriate.

Psychiatrists (specially qualified and experienced doctors) and *psychiatric nurses* are key figures in the area of mental health, although others, too, are increasingly involved. Every doctor is required to have a basic knowledge of psychiatry, while more recently, it has become mandatory for all nurses, including those training for the general part of the register, to spend a period of time caring for the mentally ill or handicapped.

Historically no such links between physical and mental health existed.

With the exception of such infectious diseases as leprosy or the plague, which carried with them a horrific derogation, physical illness evoked a good deal of sympathy. A child suffering from whooping cough, or a soldier with a gaping wound had obvious needs, and although for centuries, nursing care in such circumstances would have been ill informed, perhaps even downright dangerous, the need for intervention was at least recognised.

The gradual harnessing of this goodwill (through the efforts of such individuals as Florence Nightingale), culminating in the ambitious but laudable creation of a truly national and freely available health service, is an exciting and by now familiar story.

The evolution of psychiatric nursing is altogether different. For most of recorded history, individuals unfortunate enough to be psychologically disturbed have been ridiculed, persecuted or punished. Symptoms were seen as being due to 'the wrath of the gods', and often explained by reference to *witchcraft*. For many centuries large numbers of people, many of whom must have been mentally ill, were burned at the stake, lest as agents of the devil, their evil influences be allowed to spread.

Enlightenment was slow. By the end of the 18th century, William Tuke had founded the York Retreat, based on 'moral' treatment, which forbade the use of punishment, while encouraging kindness, understanding and a routine job of work. Such establishments, however, were rare.

But although society began to acknowledge responsibility for the mentally infirm, little was done to make psychiatric nursing respectable. Typically, large asylums were built far out in the country, to keep those poor unfortunates well away from the major centres of population. This, together with a poorly developed transport system and a total lack of knowledge regarding suitable treatments, usually meant 'lunatics', thus sent away, quickly lost touch with their families. The inmates tended to live out the rest of their lives within the introverted confines of these largely self-sufficient institutions.

As a consequence, relatives, suspecting that a family member might be mentally ill, put off seeking advice until the last possible minute, when often it was already too late to effect a recovery. This confirmed relatives' worst fears and increased pessimism.

Even as recently as the Second World War, the philosophy of caring for the insane had changed little. While it seems safe to assume that only a minority of staff ever indulged in direct acts of cruelty, the rest stood back and adopted an attitude of benign surveillance. Staff were described as attendants, acted like warders and presumably felt little affinity towards those nurses who toiled with the physically sick.

From these historical beginnings, perhaps, spring the unfortunate stereotypes of the highly skilled, overworked, 'angels' in the general hospitals, and the psychiatric nurse who sits around, doing little or nothing all day. Such myths, to some extent, remain with us even today.

The post-war years heralded the birth of the National Health Service, the introduction of several drugs which proved successful in diminishing many psychiatric symptoms, and eventually, the passing of the much liberalised Mental Health Acts (England and Wales 1959, Scotland 1960). The attendants have become nurses, the asylums are hospitals and 'insanity' is acknowledged as an illness.

Before going on to explore the role of the nurse in treating the mentally ill, it should be mentioned that a body of opinion exists that believes it is not helpful to medicalise mental disorders, or label such individuals as sick. This view will be looked at more closely in Chapter 20.

THE NURSE AND THE PSYCHIATRICALLY DISTURBED

Julie, aged 19, is half-way through her general nurse training. At her initial interview, she was surprised to discover that she would be required to spend part of her training in a psychiatric hospital. She was uncertain of how she felt about this, but rapidly relegated all thoughts on the subject to the back of her mind.

Now, however, Julie is due to start her psychiatric module, and her original doubts are resurfacing. Any general orientated nurse arriving, perhaps unwillingly, on a psychiatric ward, is likely to be filled with trepidation.

How will she react to mentally ill patients, or they to her? What special skills can she observe in her psychiatrically trained colleagues, and can she emulate them? Will she be able to spot a job of work that has to be done? If she gets it wrong, will she do irreparable damage?

Her first baptism to the world of the mentally ill will be on either an acute admission or long-term ward and will be different to anything she will have previously experienced. Consequently, she may be both apprehensive and excited.

Along with the perhaps more familiar psychogeriatric wards these areas make up the typical psychiatric hospital and Julie may be interested in observing her mentally trained colleagues function in all three situations.

Acute admission ward

These wards accommodate a wide variety of individuals for comparatively short periods of time. Males and females frequently share the same facilities; most patients will be up and about, with the accent on intensive treatment and early discharge. Some patients will spend only a few weeks in such a ward, before going home, never to return. Some may be discharged apparently well, only to be re-admitted on numerous other occasions.

Jimmy has been coming into hospital for 9 of his 24 years. A product of a one-parent family, Jimmy frequently fights with his mother, who, though finding him a handful, visits regularly. His behaviour is often impulsive, and he has been in trouble with the police. He has had many jobs, but has been unemployed for some time.

A nurse is in charge of the group therapy Jimmy attends daily. Here Jimmy can say what he likes, but physical violence is not allowed. Frequently the nurse says nothing for long intervals, but may intervene to ask a question, sum up what has been going on, or tentatively to offer an interpretation.

At other times of the day, Jimmy's impulsive approach to life cannot be allowed to go unchecked. Society has rules, and if Jimmy is to succeed, he must learn to abide by them. Clearly-defined limits have been set on certain aspects of his behaviour. He must arrive at group meetings on time, his record player must not disrupt the television programme favoured by the majority and he cannot entice the more acutely disturbed patients to leave the ward.

Should he break these rules, the consequences have been agreed by Jimmy, the psychiatrist and the nurse. Sanctions, such as a veto on the lunchtime playing of music, restrictions on the number of visits he is allowed to make to the local cafe, or a temporary ban on his daily table tennis games with the charge nurse, have to be applied. This calls for a consistent and undoubtedly, an authoritarian approach from the nurse in charge.

Jimmy is very immature and relatively naive for a young man of 24. Before an interview, a family wedding, or even a trip to an unfamiliar store, he frequently requires to rehearse the likely sequence of events, using the nurse as either a critic or a model.

Julie, by observing the nursing care of only one patient, has seen psychiatric nurses adopt a number of roles, as befits the circumstances. They are the *therapist* — penetrating and astute; *the parent* — firm but kindly intentioned; *the teacher* — patiently instructive.

At this stage, Julie may feel ill-equipped to don such a multitude of hats, but all are entirely legitimate.

Long-term wards

We have seen how, until recent times, the prognosis for any individual entering a psychiatric hospital tended to be unfavourable. Consequently, large wards, catering for many patients of long standing, were commonplace. These wards have been reduced both in size and number, as medication, and a more positive attitude, have allowed many previously considered hopeless cases to be transferred to the community.

Nevertheless, the fact that many mental disorders tend to recur, and that some patients have been in hospital for over 60 years, does mean that a smaller, but definite demand for long-term accommodation continues to exist. Nowadays, such areas are usually redesignated **rehabilitation**, wards. This change in terminology hints at a more optimistic approach and surely renders obsolete the custodial attitudes of the past.

Alec has been in hospital since the 1930s and is a familiar figure in the neighbourhood: a visitor to hospital will be guided into a parking lot by Alec, strangers will be directed to the destination of their choice by Alec and, come a winter's evening, visiting concert parties or entertainers can be sure of an eloquent speech of appreciation, from Alec.

Alec's problems are not life-threatening, although he requires a fair degree of care and attention. Left to himself he would pose no threat to the public. Yet Alec's standards are not like our own: he forgets to change his underclothes; he may elect to wear a heavy overcoat in the height of summer, or greet a visiting dignitary with his fly fully open. This is socially inappropriate and can be misinterpreted, leaving strangers frightened and Alec, in turn, rejected and despondent.

Alec sometimes requires a gentle prod in the right direction, while at other times, he needs more direct instruction. He may in the future be considered suitable for behaviour therapy, or a token economy scheme (see Ch. 7) which could involve the nurse directly in the role of therapist. In the meantime, the roles of teacher and parent are given full rein.

Psychogeriatric wards

In psychiatric hospitals, these wards make up an ever increasing percentage of the total. Patients here are sometimes described as belonging to one of three groups.

Some people, who just happen to be past retirement age, will develop psychiatric illnesses indistinguishable from those seen in others of a younger age group.

Others will have grown old there. Patients who seem destined to spend a large part of their lives in institutions will eventually reach the age when they can most suitably be accommodated in a psychogeriatric ward.

The third and largest group will suffer from psychiatric complaints directly associated with the ageing process — usually some form of *dementia*.

Here the psychiatric nurse may function in a more traditional, 'nursing' manner.

> Mrs Gray's immediate needs are obvious. She requires to be dressed, fed and kept clean. Her only wish is to visit her mother, whom she insists lives 'just around the corner', but who in reality, has been dead for over 30 years.
>
> Mrs Gray will not be 'cured' — a term seldom used in psychiatry — but nursing interventions may help arrest, or slow down the rate of deterioration.

The psychogeriatric patient will be discussed more fully in Chapter 14.

How does Julie fit into this? With no psychiatric experience, how can she be expected to cope?

This is an important misconception. Julie may never have been to a psychiatric hospital, but she certainly has experience.

She may have nursed a middle-aged man following a myocardial infarction. His anxiety will almost definitely have been a prominent feature. In the obstetric wards, postnatal depression will have been seen, while on occasion, more serious disorders like puerperal psychosis may have been encountered.

The acute confusional state, frequently due to withdrawal from alcohol (delirium tremens), may be observed in a surgical ward, while some of the Saturday night regulars at the accident and emergency department will have alcohol or personality problems.

Less dramatic, but nevertheless relevant, is the fact that almost everyone admitted to hospital will experience *heightened anxiety*, often serious enough to disrupt their normal patterns of interacting. Julie in her own state of uncertainty should be able to appreciate this, and may well feel she has more in common with some of her patients than with the more experienced staff.

There is a comforting temptation to draw a very firm line in our imagination, separating the relatively small number of psychiatrically disturbed individuals, from the rest of us, to whom we ascribe perfect sanity. This is a basic, but serious mistake. *There is no dividing line!* Everyone is capable of developing extreme anxiety, of behaving eccentrically or of feeling desperately low. It's all a matter of degree: the most well-balanced of individuals will have areas of vulnerability; the most maladjusted, areas where they function adequately.

A vital first lesson for Julie will only be understood once she has discarded this 'them and us' attitude to mental functioning and adopted the concept that everyone can be found somewhere on the same mental health/mental illness continuum (Fig. 1.1).

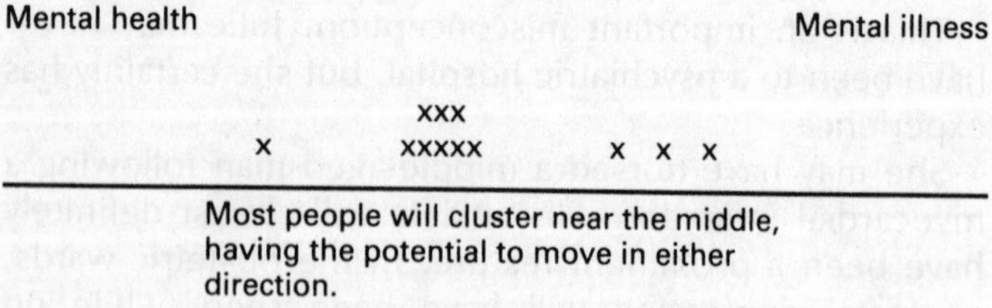

Mental health   Mental illness

```
                    xxx
          x         xxxxx        x   x   x
```
Most people will cluster near the middle, having the potential to move in either direction.

Fig. 1.1 Mental health/mental illness continuum

Individuals will move along the continuum from day to day, some may remain close to the health end, others completely the opposite. Most people will cluster near the middle, having the potential to move in either direction, depending on a variety of current stresses and individual predispositions.

UNCONSCIOUS MOTIVATION AND TRANSFERENCE

If Julie has ever suffered from glandular fever or appendicitis in the past, this in no way interferes with her ability to recognise the condition in others, or subsequently, to care compassionately for anyone so afflicted. In fact, it seems reasonable to assume that her inside knowledge and painful memories may actually enhance her standard of care in such circumstances.

But what if Julie is chronically anxious in the presence of her superiors, or entrenched in a love/hate relationship with her mother? Would she notice, or place any great emphasis on similar traits in one of her patients?

The amount of significance she places on the information that someone in her care customarily consumes 4 pints of beer daily, may differ, depending on whether she is teetotal, or whether *she* usually drinks 6!

The realisation that care staff are not uncomplicated, rational human beings comes eventually to everyone involved in psychiatry, and can be hard to take. This lack of rationality frequently complicates the nurse-patient relationship.

Julie may be flattered that one patient has taken an instant liking to her, but puzzled that another physically trembles when approached by sister or the psychiatrist. If she is entirely honest, she will admit to having positive feelings to some patients, while others, she may find difficult to like.

Yet all this can occur within a few hours of her arrival

on the ward! Closer investigation often reveals that such instant feelings are based on other than a realistic appraisal of the facts. A ward sister may trigger off reactions previously felt towards an authoritarian parent; a young patient may rekindle feelings of jealousy which originated towards a more successful brother or sister in childhood.

This tendency to attribute feelings and attitudes felt towards some significant person in the past, to someone in a current interpersonal relationship, is called *transference*. It is even more important as a feature of psychotherapy, where such transference between patient and therapist is considered essential for a successful outcome.

Anyone wishing to use their personality to help or understand others, must realise the power of *unconscious motivation* and appreciate the fact that all of us are influenced by desires and instincts outside our recognition or control.

MEETING THE PATIENTS

Having established that psychiatric patients are not a race apart, Julie would not be surprised to find that most of them are up and about. Some may be obviously depressed; others may, through discussion, reveal some rather bizarre ideas, but others still, will show no obvious abnormality whatsoever.

The various skills required to deal with specific situations will be considered in Chapter 3, but Julie cannot be expected immediately to become a carbon copy of her psychiatrically trained colleagues. This is not in itself a disadvantage. Many patients will welcome what they consider to be a less threatening atmosphere engendered by the newer arrivals and may choose to confide in them.

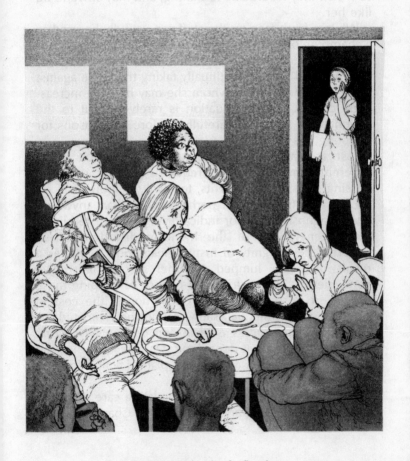

Meeting the patients for the first time . . .

Some patients, consciously or unconsciously, see the nurse as a representative of the caring, clean-cut world to which they would like to belong, and may strive to be like her.

While a fresh face on the staff can usefully be used as a champion of patients' rights, the new nurse must guard against *over identifying* with them. When this happens, she may find herself continually taking their side against other staff members of whom she may become increasingly critical. Such a situation is rarely helpful to the patients and she must carefully explore her reasons for adopting this role.

Just as Jimmy, Alec and Mrs Gray exhibit vastly different symptomatology, requiring a wide range of nursing skills, other patients, too, will be individuals.

In psychiatric nursing, perhaps more than anywhere else, diagnosis is a poor indicator of the care required. Many generations of the mentally disordered have suffered the indignity of institutionalisation, partly as a result of being lumped together for administrative convenience. The cost in hard finance of keeping these people in hospital must be phenomenal; the cost in wasted human potential, sadly, cannot be estimated.

The nursing process is alive and well in psychiatric nursing, offering as it does, long overdue individualised care for the patients, as well as a plan of action for staff such as Julie.

Taking a nursing history and formulating care plans are specialised tasks and are the subject of Chapter 2.

SUGGESTED READING

The following list can be used for general reference purposes for topics mentioned throughout the book. Texts pertaining to more specific issues will be recommended at the end of the relevant chapter.

Henderson D K, Gillespie R D 1969 Textbook of psychiatry, 10th edn. Oxford University Press, Oxford

Maddison D, Kellehear K J 1982 Psychiatric nursing, 5th edn. Churchill Livingstone, Edinburgh

Mitchell R G 1983 Breakdown, Commonsense psychiatry for nurses. Nursing Times Publications, Macmillan Journals, London

The nursing process
Patient profile
First stage nursing history
Second stage nursing history
Interviewing the relatives
Care planning
Implementing the care plan
Evaluation

2

Systematic psychiatric nursing care

The need to treat patients as *individuals* is gradually becoming more widely acknowledged in all branches of nursing. The concept of the 'appendix in bed four' is being replaced by an appreciation of the fact that a patient is more than merely a diagnosis. This is particularly true of the psychiatrically disordered.

In one sense it could be argued that the term 'appendicitis' gives us a fair idea of the symptoms and treatment experienced by anyone with that condition. Similarly, the outcome for such a person can be estimated with some certainty. The same cannot be said for a psychiatric disorder such as schizophrenia.

> John has been in hospital for almost 50 years. He is neglectful of his appearance and strongly dislikes women. In anticipation of starting his work with the hospital porter, he gets up at 6 o'clock every morning, steadfastly refusing even to take days off or holidays. On occasion recently he has been incontinent of urine.
>
> Jennifer shares John's diagnostic label but few of his therapeutic needs. At 22 years of age, she elects to spend most of her time lying in bed, to the obvious displeasure of her widowed mother. Physically attractive, she has no shortage of male admirers and dabbles half-heartedly in prostitution during the less acute phases of her illness.

Clearly John and Jennifer have little in common. Although both may be in need of psychiatric help, their treatment goals will be very different.

Any comparison between a physical condition and a psychiatric one, however superficial, will be abhorrent to some people. They will claim that this leads to unnecessarily ascribing illness to people who in effect really have 'problems in living'. They may fear that this signifies a slavish adherence to the 'medical model' of psychiatry, which tends to underplay the importance of social, cultural and psychological factors in psychiatric disorder.

Who, they ask, has the right to say that Jennifer is sick?

THE NURSING PROCESS

The nursing process however does not imply subservience to the medical or any other model. It can be applied wherever nursing is carried out. Only such an approach which emphasises the fact that each person is a unique individual with unique needs and potentials can hope to be successful.

Julie, fresh from her general ward, will be familiar with the nursing process and its claim to facilitate systematic, personalised nursing care. She will recognise its relevance to psychiatry.

The nursing process is not without its detractors, many of whom are psychiatric nurses. They claim that its four accepted stages of *assessment, planning, implementation* and *evaluation* have always been practised automatically by anyone with even a modicum of commonsense and represent merely an attempt to render as scientific something they have been doing for many years. The additional paperwork they resent, deeming it unnecessary. The disordered mind, they claim, is too complex to be shackled by any administrative framework.

They may have a point. The possessor of a disturbed mind is indeed a complex being who must be approached with a great deal of flexibility. However, the nursing process seems ideally suited to provide this flexibility.

The psychiatric nursing history/patient profile

In order to formulate a realistic nursing programme for the Johns and Jennifers of this world, a detailed, all-encompassing nursing history must be obtained.

Crow (1979) suggests: 'If insufficient time or trouble is taken over assessment, fewer patient problems will be identified. This means that the second stage: that of constructing a care plan to assist the patient with his or her identified problem, will not be as comprehensive as it might have been.'

It is vital that such a history be more than an instant snapshot of the management problems at that moment when admission to hospital becomes necessary. The term '*patient profile*' implies a more ongoing process of assessment, culminating in a fluent 'identikit' of the patient that is both objective and meaningful.

It should be remembered that most potential patients present for a psychiatric admission in an orderly manner as a result of a previously made appointment. However, some may be sent by the courts, admitted against their will, or they may arrive in a state of great excitement or depression. Clearly the circumstances surrounding their presentation for treatment will greatly influence the depth of the nursing history that can be obtained at this time.

Julie may be experienced in taking histories and will almost certainly have admitted many patients. The principles with which she is familiar remain applicable.

In even the most dramatic admission a certain amount of paperwork is necessary. It is essential to be able to identify the patient and this would at the very least involve the recording of his name and address. Further related information such as the name of the next of kin, the date of birth and the religion are important and should normally be written down as a precursor to the profile proper.

Anyone being admitted to hospital is likely to be anxious and may react unpredictably. Some will withdraw into a shell while others may chatter nineteen to the dozen. Few however will communicate meaningfully until they feel able to trust the nurse to whom they are expected to bare their soul.

McFarlane & Castledine (1982) speak of first stage and second stage nursing histories. Although they refer mainly to physically ill patients, the principle holds good.

The first stage history is an extension of what has been described above. It is essentially a fact-finding session and when dealing with patients who are not unduly disturbed, it is an integral part of the admission procedure. When circumstances demand, it may be short and hurriedly transcribed but will nevertheless form the basis for the immediate plan of action.

The second stage history, particularly with a psychiatric patient, will be far more detailed and may take a considerable time to compile. Of special interest will be details of past hospitalisations, any apparent precipitating factors and the patient's own account of his problems. We will want to identify the significant people in his life and note any traumatic childhood experiences. Particularly relevant may be how the patient's present behaviour or level of functioning compares with his past performances.

Mr K. presented as a quiet but polite individual, who smiled when approached by staff. He appeared to watch television a lot, preferably on his own. He got up at 5.30 each morning.
Such a history may appear insignificant until Mr K.'s past lifestyle is considered. It transpired that he was normally a

jovial type who was unable to sit around for long and enjoyed a boisterous good time with a wide variety of acquaintances. Usually he would rise for breakfast at around 7.45 a.m.

Only by considering Mr K. before and after he sought help can we recognise the extent to which his illness has changed his way of life. This change would be borne in mind when formulating his care plan.

Early morning wakening, a decrease in energy and a wish to be alone are a combination of symptoms which tends to occur together in many patients and would hint at a medical diagnosis of depression.

As many signs and symptoms occur and recur in recognisable sequences which directly influence the planning of nursing care, the nurse may find it useful to carry a checklist (possibly mental) to which she can refer.

During the initial contact between nurse and patient, the nurse may find it particularly rewarding to observe the following:

General appearance. This may range from normal, through to unkempt to the frankly bizarre. Mannerisms or stereotyped movements, if present, may be significant, as is the apparent general health of the patient.

Speech. Important here is the *rate* of speech which may be accelerated to such an extent as to be incoherent, or slowed down to the point of mutism.

By listening to the *content* of the speech, the nurse may gain some insight into her patient's problems. He may state that he wishes he was dead or that he is Jesus Christ. He may voice his fear of cats or his belief that he is being pursued by an oriental assassin.

The general rate of activity will mirror the rate of speech, while any obviously unusual pattern should be noted.

Concentration. It is common for the ability to concentrate to be diminished, so the length of the attention span is an observation worth making.

The mood. The mood, or as it is known in psychiatry, the *affect*, is capable of great variation in any one individual. Extremes of mood or emotions, or a sudden swing in either direction, may be significant, while its appropriateness to current events should be gauged.

As the nurse/patient relationship develops, these observations, particularly should they have changed since admission, remain important. However, as the second stage history is gradually compiled, still further areas can be explored.

A rough estimate can be made of the patient's level of **intelligence**. Mental illness is no respector of intellectual ability and wide variations will be discovered. If it is considered necessary, a formal intelligence test may be administered by the team psychologist.

Memory too can be assessed with specific attention being paid to poor or patchy recall. Confabulation, the unconscious filling in of memory gaps with a seemingly suitable explanation, and a marked deterioration of recent memory alongside adequate long-term recall, are examples of relatively common memory malfunctions.

Insight, the recognition by the patient that he is ill, may or may not be present and this will affect the care plan. Someone who acknowledges that he is unwell is more likely to take some responsibility for his own recovery.

Important though the aforementioned observations may be, they are worthless if they represent only the subjective whim of the nurse. Her role is to observe objectively what she sees, preferably using a minimum of medical jargon. Speech if possible should be recorded verbatim and only behaviour actually witnessed should be written down.

Statements such as 'hallucinating freely this a.m.' tell us little. In contrast 'Looking out of the window, shaking his fist and swearing loudly at the apparently empty lawn at 10.30 this morning,' is better, but whoever reads it must draw their own conclusions or investigate further.

The nurse who observes meticulously will discover much that is important, but this is not adequate history taking.

The patient and his significant friends or relatives must be encouraged to contribute actively. Family history, scholastic achievements and childhood illnesses may be reported by anyone, but seemingly trivial questions may sometimes reveal widely divergent viewpoints.

> Jimmy, a young man in hospital for the first time, described his father as 'cold and aloof, a rather frightening figure,' while his mother said his father was a hard worker who loved his children.
> Both may have been correct.
> Jimmy described their neighbour, a policeman, as 'a Satanist, in league with the devil,' whereas his mother said he was 'a quiet man, who minded his own business.'
> This could be significant.

While a formal interview has the advantage of speed and consistency of questions, some psychiatric patients will find it too threatening. If the nurse, too, is unsure of herself, the more detailed second stage history may best be accomplished as a *participant observer*.

During daily activities on the ward, at occupational therapy, or in walks in the hospital grounds, Julie, as she gradually gains confidence, can steer the conversation in directions she believes important. By actually working alongside the patient, valuable spontaneity, which may otherwise be absent, is encouraged. The skill of asking open-ended questions, which require more than a one word answer, can best be practised in such a setting.

Interviewing the relatives

The relatives however should normally be interviewed in a conventional manner in private. It is what they will expect and lends to the proceedings an air of formality which is appropriate.

Before commencing the interview, the nurse should remind herself quickly of what is already known about the patient. This she can achieve by glancing through his medical case notes and the partially completed nursing history. Having thus refreshed her memory, she must endeavour to put the information to the back of her mind so that she can conduct the proceedings as objectively as possible.

During the interview, privacy is essential. Both participants should be comfortably seated fairly close together with no artificial barrier such as a desk between them. In order to gain the wholehearted support of the interviewee, the nurse should explain the importance of the information in planning the most suitable nursing care. When appropriate, the relative may be involved in this planning and should usually be made aware of the broad aims of the treatment.

The role of the nurse is to facilitiate communication by gently directing conversation towards sensitive areas, without apparently dismissing any trivia that the relative may consider important.

A safe, encouraging atmosphere can sometimes be fostered with only a minimal preamble. Non-verbal communication such as eye contact, a smile or the occasional friendly grunt can indicate that the nurse is interested. If this is interspersed with the occasional 'really' or 'please, do tell me more,' information may flow freely.

By reversing this technique, a skilled interviewer can tactfully discourage a train of conversation by purposely discontinuing eye contact.

From the onset, the nurse will have some idea of the themes which have to be explored. She may decide to use a standard questionnaire on which responses can be written or ticked, or may favour a much less-structured approach. Either way, if the history is to highlight potential nursing problems and form the basis for planning their solution, recording must be accurate and complete.

Information received from relatives or friends, like reports from the patient, form only part of the picture. Details acquired in this way may be unwittingly biased or deliberately distorted. No one can be completely neutral when dealing with the intimate problems of a loved one. For instance, this fact is widely recognised by members of the medical profession, who as a result, never treat their own families. Nurses may be surprised at the extent to which some relatives can rationalise or minimise bizarre conduct in the patient. At times this may even raise doubts as to just how strong is their own grip on reality.

Others may plan a little deceit.

It must be to society's everlasting shame, that it has consistently failed to make adequate provision for those who accept the onerous task of caring for a relative in the community. On occasion, carers may feel they need to exaggerate the extent of the patient's problem in order to give themselves the respite, which should be theirs by right. This may result in the patient who never quite lives up to the fearful reputation which preceded him to hospital.

Conversely, family loyalty may mean that some factors about the patient may be deliberately withheld. Eccentricities, considered by the interviewee to be shameful or ridiculous, may go unreported.

Consequently, information about such things as incontinence, homosexuality or a liking for tomato ketchup on his cornflakes may become obvious only after the patient arrives on the ward.

Some people will present themselves for admission unaccompanied. This is contrary to the accepted cultural practice and should be noted as potentially significant. It is easy for us to refer glibly to relatives as if assuming that all patients below a certain age automatically reside with two stable parents. This stereotyping may continue with the assumption that marriage and parenthood will follow, thus perpetuating the ready supply of caring relations. While true for a large percentage of the population, doubtless we can all think of exceptions. This picture is unarguably idealised and can never be applied to the population as a whole.

More recently, the number of divorces has increased, single-parent families seem to be more common and in some circles, intimate relationships appear much less permanent than we have been traditionally conditioned to believe.

The potential psychiatric patient may well be a product of such a background. An unsettled childhood may have somehow predisposed him to later breakdown or, on the other hand, his past conduct may have been sufficiently outrageous to alienate him from his family. He may have 'drifted' towards the anonymity of life in a big city centre as his illness progressed, a feature common to many disturbed young people.

Whatever the explanation, a caring relative will not be available in every case and additional information must be sought elsewhere. Social workers, landladies, police or cohabitees may be able to help, but can only be approached if the patient gives consent.

Whatever the sources, the patient profile will eventually take shape. Problems or potential problems will appear, treatment priorities will emerge and care planning can proceed.

Care planning

Care plans, carefully complied and updated as frequently as necessary, are a valuable communication tool. Based on the nursing problems, highlighted during the history taking, they ensure the consistent application of individualised care.

In order to facilitate implementation and subsequent

evaluation, the plans should be written in an unambiguous fashion with the objectives being readily measurable and realistically attainable. When appropriate, a time limit for reaching the objectives should be fixed.

> Mary arrived reluctantly in hospital in a very emaciated condition. On completion of her nursing history it transpired that she weighed only 39.4 kg and was caught up in an extremely complicated love/hate relationship with both her mother and younger sister.

A sample of the objectives chosen for her was:

a. within 3 weeks, she would sit at the table and eat a full meal
b. she would reach her 'target' weight by the end of August
c. she would develop a more satisfactory relationship with her mother and sister.

Objectives *a* and *b* seem reasonable and are clear cut. By the end of 3 weeks she will either be sitting at the table eating a meal, or she will not. The success or otherwise of the plan can be gauged and if necessary it can be modified.

Objective *c* is altogether less realistic. How much more satisfactory must the relationship be before the objective is reached. How long must we wait to see if the improvement will materialise? The idea is laudable, but it should be rephrased in a measurable, tangible manner.

Having set the objectives, it must be decided how best they can be met. A plan of action must be developed.

To meet objective *a* the prescribed nursing action might be:

(i) offer attractive average sized meals at each ward meal time
(ii) sit with Mary, encouraging her to eat and observing surreptitious 'dumping' of foodstuffs
(iii) reward with privileges as per agreed 'contract' — when plate is emptied.

The 'contract' referred to may have been drawn up between Mary and the member of staff primarily responsible for her care. It would involve giving Mary a reward which is valued by her on progress being achieved. Such rewards increase the likelihood of the progress being repeated or maintained.

Implementing the care plan

For the nurse, it is easy to carry out this plan and should any changes become necessary, they will be clearly written down. At any one time, therefore, she can tell at a glance if the objectives have been achieved, or if further adjustments are required.

Evaluation

If the objectives are not achieved, this may be due to one of a number of reasons:

1. the original assessment may have been faulty, e.g. Mary's lack of eating may have had a physical, rather than psychological cause.
2. the nursing action prescribed may have been unsuitable (close observation may make her more determined) or unrealistic (was the nurse sufficiently experienced to carry it out?).
3. the implementation may have been faulty — some nurses observed closely and gave rewards when earned; others didn't bother.
4. the expected outcome may have been unrealistic; after all, 3 weeks is a comparatively short time for such a radical change.

In other words, failure to meet an objective would demand a reappraisal of each stage of the nursing process and the efficiency with which it was carried out. The evaluation thus evolves into a fresh assessment and the circular nature of the nursing process is apparent.

Nursing histories, when complete, may contain a great deal of personal information and due recognition of this must be made when deciding how and where they should be stored. Care plans, however, to be effective must be updated regularly and be readily accessible to all members of the staff. While storage and retrieval systems will vary from hospital to hospital, some sort of 'Kardex' arrangement generally fits the bill.

The value to the patient of planned systematic care must by now be obvious. This alone should atone for any extra paper work accrued by the staff.

For Julie, it will be a godsend. In strange surroundings, anything that is familiar will be welcome. Nursing histories and care plans she will understand. The fear of the unknown will be partly eclipsed and the question frantically asked by so many newcomers to psychiatric nursing, 'but what do we actually *do*?' will be less necessary.

In the nursing chapters that follow, it can be assumed that the approach outlined above will be the one that is recommended.

REFERENCES

Crow J 1979 Assessment. In: Kratz C (ed) The nursing process. Baillière Tindall, London
McFarlane J, Castledine G 1982 A guide to the practice of nursing using the nursing process. C V Mosby, London

The patient who is suicidal
The patient who is overactive or excited
The patient who is violent or aggressive
The patient who is confused
The patient who is incontinent
The patient who refuses to eat
The patient who is institutionalised

3

Psychiatric nursing — guidelines to care

Whatever the patient's specific problem, individual, systematic nursing care must remain the approach of choice. Nevertheless, it would be foolhardy to deny that many different patients can produce behaviour which is similar. This chapter looks at the broad principles of nursing care in some of the situations most likely to be encountered by the nurse in psychiatry.

THE PATIENT WHO IS SUICIDAL

Julie may find the thought of suicide abhorrent. Culturally and religiously the taking of one's own life has always been taboo, and until recently, even to attempt to do so was a criminal offence. Nurses, traditionally dedicated to the concept of cure, may feel threatened by the thought of a patient deliberately setting out to kill himself. After all many of their previous patients will have gone to great lengths to stay alive.

It is a fact that a proportion of psychiatric patients at any one time is likely to be contemplating suicide. Some will get round to attempting it, while a tiny minority may actually succeed.

People try to kill themselves for many reasons. They may be hearing voices giving them instructions to do so, or they may be responding to adverse environmental factors (e.g. redundancy, bereavement or bankruptcy). Some may feel deep guilt or remorse as a result of a psychological disorder (alcoholism) or a physical complaint (syphilis), but the majority will probably feel engulfed in deep gloom or despondency for which they can offer no explanation. The intense misery of this group means that they are the ones most likely to commit the successful suicide.

Features suggestive of suicidal intentions

Certain features in the nursing history, occurring separately or in combination, should alert the nurse to the possibility that her patient may be suicidal:

a. a history of past suicidal attempts.
b. pessimistic or gloomy utterances: the French term, a cri de coeur, (a cry from the heart) describes the phenomenon, supposed to be widespread, of the potential suicide letting slip his intentions, however indirectly. Failure to interpret this cry for help may result in a preventable death
c. giving away valued possessions
d. age — middle-aged to elderly
e. sex — male, rather than female
f. a history of sleep disturbance, usually involving early morning wakening
g. an apparent lightening of the mood after a period of intense gloom.
h. a successful suicide by a significant family member.

In addition, the myth that people who talk about killing themselves never do so, must be totally repudiated. Anyone voicing suicidal thoughts must be taken very, very seriously indeed.

Principles of care

The principles governing the nursing care of a suicidal patient are:

1. maintain life and prevent injury
2. ensure adequate nourishment and personal hygiene
3. environmental manipulation
4. assist with medical procedures.

Maintaining life and preventing injury

Patients who are acutely suicidal will be incapable of maintaining their life and are likely to do anything they can to end it. Some may have been admitted compulsorily to hospital following a serious suicide attempt or after a request from their GP or a relative who can no longer monitor them confidently at home. Many others will have entered hospital voluntarily, either in order to gain relief from their crippling despondency, or because they may vaguely realise that here, others will try to stop what they themselves can no longer prevent.

Either way, the hospital has temporarily assumed a large degree of responsibility for the patient's well-being. This is recognised by the staff and the relatives, even when not acknowledged by the patient.

One consequence of this awesome responsibility is the fact that no one discipline can formulate the treatment plan. On admission, and after brief consultation between the psychiatrist, nurse and relevant others, a patient may be designated as being a high suicide risk. His care must be planned accordingly.

Traditionally at such a time, the nurse is asked to provide strict, *24 hour surveillance* on the patient in her charge. During the acute phase this may best be achieved by briefly confining the patient to bed. On admission, a careful check on the patient's belongings must be carried out in his presence. Any obviously

dangerous article must be removed with a brief explanation and a reassurance that it will be returned should
it be required. Razors, nail files and manicure sets come
into this category. Potentially lethal items such as drugs
are easily secreted by a desperate patient, while the
damage that can be inflicted by everyday objects like
knitting needles must not be overlooked.

This meticulous examination of their property may be
offensive to some people, but is generally less so if they
are encouraged to assist. The patient's presence is
required as a common courtesy, as a safeguard against
subsequent claims that items have disappeared and so
that the nurse can explore the reason for any suspicious
articles being hidden.

Many nurses will not enjoy this violation of her
patient's personal property, but apart from actually
saving a life, she may, by her thoroughness, impart a
message of caring. For someone whose sense of unworthiness may be threatening to overpower him, this
may be the first tangible sign that someone is interested
enough to care if he lives or dies.

Patients, even if confined to bed, should be allowed
up every 24 hours for supervised bathing. At this time the
opportunity should be taken to remake the bed,
checking once again for potentially lethal objects.
Hanging is a relatively common method of suicide, and
dressing gown cords, neckties and belts should be
removed or accounted for. The nurse has an important
responsibility to see that all *drugs* prescribed and administered are actually swallowed, but caches of uncon-
sumed medication should be sought at this time.

Supervised bathing or having a witness in the toilet will
be extremely embarrassing for many people although
they may not have the energy to complain. Nurses like
Julie may also find this task distasteful, but must take
great care not to show it. Any indication that she finds
the patient disgusting would fuel his feelings of dispair.

Nurses who relax their vigilance at this point because of mistaken kindness, may be punished unmercifully by a preventable death.

It is impossible to observe anyone closely for a prolonged period of time without making him aware of it. It is pointless to try. Patients should be told truthfully that they are being observed, and if necessary, why they are being observed. This frequently makes the nurse's task easier, since it dispenses with the need for deceit.

If observing for any length of time, the nurse will find it advantageous if she can involve her patient in a game of draughts, dominoes or in discussion, but this may not be possible. If the patient is deeply depressed, he may ignore all friendly overtures, preferring to sit in silence. This means that the nurse must guard against becoming too involved in a book or other such diversion, to the detriment of the task on hand.

The regime described above is time-consuming, dehumanising and justifiable only in that it saves lives. Sooner or later, some relaxation must thankfully take place, hopefully as a result of multidisciplinary deliberations.

Some authorities believe that a similar success rate can be achieved by employing a less repressive approach and it is common to confine patients merely to pyjamas and dressing gown. They believe that the patient's self-esteem will increase if more emphasis is placed on establishing trust. While such an aim is laudable, it presupposes that the patient is in a state of mind to handle such trust. This cannot be guaranteed. In any case, the hospital must never abdicate its responsibility lightly, since even one preventable suicide is unacceptable.

When patients are up and about this undoubtedly puts an extra strain on staff. Lotions, drugs and innumerable sharp objects are now potentially within reach and must continually be accounted for. Nurses should be constantly aware of their patients' whereabouts and must be able to furnish a description of their dress and appearance in the event of them leaving the hospital.

The responsibility for maintaining life and preventing injury is not the nurse's alone.

The traditional psychiatric hospital had several *architectural features* geared towards the prevention of suicide. Staircases were built in such a way as to prevent people jumping over the bannisters, fires were well guarded and windows were too small to get through easily. Bath taps were removable, or could only be controlled by keys. These features are usually considered unattractive, and are gradually disappearing in the latest attempts to de-institutionalise our institutions. Efforts aimed at making our hospitals more homely must rightly be applauded, but a word of caution is required.

Architects and planners must continue to be guided by features other than aestheticism. The safety of the patient must remain a priority.

Ensuring adequate nourishment and personal hygiene

If close, rather detatched observation was the nurse's only role in dealing with a suicidal patient, she would find it less than rewarding. This is plainly not so. Maintaining life must admittedly be the number one priority, but nursing interventions will also be required in other, almost as important areas.

Because of lethargy, a feeling of unworthiness, or in a rather clumsy attempt to kill themselves, some patients will *refuse to eat*. They may believe that they are too poor to buy the food which they are convinced must be paid for, or they may think it tastes unpleasant and decide that it has been poisoned. Patients who refuse to eat are discussed in greater depth later on in this chapter.

The nurse by her caring yet firm attitude must make it plain that her patient is far too important to be allowed to starve himself to death. In a life-threatening situation nasogastric feeding would have to be considered, but thankfully in practice, this is seldom required.

Similarly, someone determined to kill himself will not appreciate the need to *wash or bathe* regularly. This is unfortunate. A bath or general 'freshen up' makes the individual feel better, and of course, to be socially clean helps prevent a rebuff from fellow patients, who if they were to complain of his unkempt or smelly state, could further shatter an already fragile self image.

In encouraging, and initially assisting the patient to bathe, the nurse should never lose sight of the fact that observed bathing may be extremely embarrassing for some people. Although sometimes inevitable, it is a fact that once such restrictions can safely be removed, an upsurge of interest in personal hygiene may quickly follow.

Environmental manipulation

An attempted or threatened suicide represents a crisis for the patient. It is also an important event for the significant others in his life. Admission to a psychiatric hospital may further exaggerate the attendant emotions. It may come as a complete surprise to a spouse, neighbour or relative that someone whom they thought they knew well could become so desperate. It may make them feel guilty.

Admission to hospital may be just what is required to focus attention on the patient's problems and to elicit help from those around him. A carefully taken nursing history may suggest that referal to a *social worker* would be appropriate, and problems with housing, family or finance may be ventilated.

Kate (62 years old) was admitted following a serious suicide attempt by gassing, which was foiled purely by chance. Obese and formerly of good spirits, she had increasingly withdrawn from her social acquaintances. At length, she had become almost a recluse in the single-roomed, rented flat where she lived along.

After treatment with ECT it became possible for Kate to return home, with her only relatives, two nieces, promising to keep an eye on her. It was arranged that she attend a lunch club and she has agreed to help out at at a local Sunday School crèche. It is to be hoped that the crippling isolation, which came so close to overwhelming her, can now be kept at bay.

The nurse plays a crucial part in maintaining an appropriate atmosphere in the ward. Exaggerated joviality or back slapping hilarity is certainly inappropriate. Forced participation in games or activities may also be counter-productive. A non-threatening, mildly cheerful environment is the ideal, with patients being encouraged to take part in friendly conversation or non-competitive diversion once they feel up to it.

Assisting in medical procedures

In Chapter 6, physical methods of treatment will be discussed. It will highlight the important therapeutic contribution of drugs and ECT. The nurse must ensure that the patient is given the prescribed quantity of the correct drug at the time specified by the doctor. In particular she must be certain that they are swallowed and not saved for consumption in bulk during a subsequent suicide bid.

Nursing care — before, during and after ECT — requires a high standard of skill in both general and psychiatric nursing, and may be welcomed by Julie as being at least partly familiar.

If suicide occurs

With the best will in the world, suicide cannot be totally eradicated. Occasionally, a former or current patient may succeed in killing himself, either at home or in hospital. Such an event can be shattering.

Feelings of anger, guilt, impotence and genuine grief may well up in relatives, staff and other patients. Relatives may openly accuse hospital staff of negligence, and the nurse may wonder if in fact they are right. Other patients, too, may feel they should have been able to help. They may also be vaguely frightened by the realisation that their own impulses and behaviour cannot automatically be rendered neutral by the all-competent nurses. There may even be some danger of one or even perhaps a spate of 'copy cat' suicide bids.

Most people will more readily accept the situation if they are able to talk openly about their emotions and reactions to a warm individual not directly involved.

Investigations should be thorough, not primarily to apportion blame (the patient is already dead) but to try to prevent a recurrence. The ward or hospital routine may have to be altered depending on what is discovered.

The maxim that anyone who really wants to kill himself will eventually succeed is meant to instil neither frustration nor complacency in nurses, but nevertheless, has some truth in it. In the unlikely event of a suicide taking place during her short module in psychiatry, the nurse need not be full of self recriminations. If she acted professionally and in good faith, she should try to put it down as a potent, if particularly gruesome, learning experience. Hopefully, a repetition will thus be avoided.

THE PATIENT WHO IS OVERACTIVE OR EXCITED

While much is written about caring for the suicidal patient, fewer guidelines exist on how the nurse should care for someone who is overactive or excited. This may be due to the fact that the unpredictability of these symptoms make hard and fast rules utterly ridiculous.

As we shall see, some individuals suffer from *both extremes* of mood and activity during their lifetime and will therefore require their care to be altered accordingly. Most commonly, an upsurge in the rate of activity accompanies a feeling of enhanced well-being and an acceleration in the rate of speech. It may occur in people who have a history of previous depressive illness.

Overactivity may also be precipitated by acute anxiety, childhood problems associated with minimal brain damage, hallucinatory experiences or physical complaints such as thyrotoxicosis. In these cases, the sense of well-being is likely to be absent and the enthusiastic zest for life is missing.

Faced with a barrage of nursing problems she may not previously have encountered, Julie will be relieved to discover that it is possible to determine a list of priorities. These include the need to ensure adequate nourishment and rest, the necessity of protecting the patient's integrity and the importance of minimising the effects of his behaviour on fellow patients.

Ensuring adequate nourishment and rest

While some patients, only marginally overactive, may greedily bolt their food in a gluttonous manner, this is likely to be short lasting. As their rate of activity increases, their concentration will diminish and they will simply not have the time for such trivialities as eating or drinking.

The use of drugs thankfully means that patients do not, as a rule, remain extremely hyperactive for more than a few days, but while they are, it is important to ensure an adequate nutritional intake.

The overactive patient, continually on the move, will not sit still long enough to eat a meal, and may even become aggressive if any attempt is made to use force. On the other hand, grapes or biscuits lying unguarded on a neighbour's locker may be surreptitiously consumed.

Suitable foods such as sausage rolls, apples or filled rolls can be left where they will be readily seen, or can be handed to the patient as he hurries past. Drinks, which should ideally be served in an unbreakable container, should be similarly offered at every turn. Much ingenuity is required if enough nourishment is to be taken, and a flexible attitude giving full consideration to any personal preference is essential. A little bit of anything they fancy, in what is potentially a life-threatening situation, will almost certainly do them good!

The extremely overactive patient will feel no need to rest, and in the past, deaths from a mixture of exhaustion and dehydration/starvation were reported. A quiet, peaceful environment, probably in a side room, dim lighting and a sympathetic nurse may encourage sleep, as will the unlikely acceptance of a warm bath or milky drink. Should he sit down and momentarily drop off, this should be counted as a blessing and he should be allowed to dose wherever he may be. If necessary, a warm blanket can be placed over him, but it it not advisable to wake him to get him into bed. Once wakened he is unlikely to fall asleep again, but as he is becoming orientated, he may more readily accept a nourishing drink which would otherwise be refused.

Protecting the patient's integrity

The bulk of overactive, excited patients eventually return to a normal level of functioning, with their insight and intellectual capacity restored. Although this is something for which we should be grateful, it does mean they may be painfully aware of their exploits when they were disturbed. Consequently, they may suffer acute embarrassment. Since we have established that many people who display these symptoms seem also to have a built-in potential for developing depression, the nurse must be aware of the possibility that the memory of recent events may precipitate an episode of low spirits.

When acutely ill, the overactive patient may be sexually uninhibited. He may dislike the restrictions imposed by his clothes and abandon them whenever possible. He may pass critical, suggestive or frankly obscene remarks to nurses or fellow patients, who if unprepared, may take offence.

He may negotiate grandiose business deals, committing himself and his family to financial agreements which he cannot afford, or may write or phone important people with whom he claims to be intimate. He may write to the press boldly sounding off about some matter which may subsequently rebound on him, causing embarrassment.

Julie will clearly be aware of her responsibility to prevent her patient from causing himself later anguish, but may be at a loss as to what she can do. His *distractability* may come to the rescue.

A patient writing a long letter advising the Chancellor of the Exchequer on the latest economic crisis will not stop if ordered to do so, but seconds later may be unable to resist telling Julie how best she should play her hand of dominoes. A patient demanding the use of the ward telephone may suddenly spot a seagull out of the corner of his eye, and immediately start to plan a campaign for feeding birds in winter. This idea, too, will be fleeting, but a crisis will have been avoided.

Long before Julie ever reaches her psychiatric module she will have been made well aware of the need for *confidentiality*. Nevertheless, this is an appropriate time to remind her. Some of her patients may be extremely funny, perhaps even providing her with a repertoire of jokes. Their behaviour may be bizzare or outrageous, but will almost certainly be interesting. At one level, Julie may feel almost cheated that her wealth of new found anecdotes cannot be repeated, but she will realise that it is essential that they are not. This can be more difficult, but even more important if her patient is well known or respected in the community or in wider society. If they are to have any chance of successfully reintegrating with their past lifestyle they must be certain that their 'secrets' are safe. The tale of how they spent several days with few clothes on, singing bawdy songs or chasing nurses round the ward, although potentially newsworthy, must remain forever untold.

Other patients

The overactive patient may interfere with his fellow patients' belongings, keep them awake at night or offend them with his lack of personal hygiene. If this continues for any length of time, a great deal of ill feeling may be engendered.

Initially, this is not so. Unless his symptoms are extreme the others may be amused at his jokes and envious of his energy. At this point any attempt by the staff to calm him down against his will may even meet with protests from the patient population who urge that we leave him alone. But it will not last.

If honest, the nurse may have to acknowledge a rising irritation, as her good intentions are continually thwarted. The same jokes wear a little thin, the repeated interfering becomes tiresome. Yet the nurse is supposedly psychologically well balanced and spends less than a third of her day on duty.

The impact on other patients, themselves hospitalised presumably because of some inability to cope, and who remain there for the whole of the 24 hours, is potentially devastating.

The sometimes conflicting nursing priorities must include the saving of the overactive patient from the wrath of the others, who in turn should be afforded the peace and privacy which is their right.

If considered to be unlikely to run away, the fitter

overactive patient may benefit from a walk in the hospital grounds or even a simple game of football. Fellow patients may also benefit from a walk, but will doubtless head off in the opposite direction!

Activities such as painting on a large surface, with big brushes and bright colours may be enjoyed, but patients, staff and property must be well protected from the paint which should be water-based.

On the other hand, anything requiring concentration or fine movements is useless and it is doubtful if it is worthwhile introducing jigsaw puzzles or Scrabble to the ward at such a time. They will merely frustrate the over-active patient who will then make it impossible for anyone else to enjoy them either.

Nursing the overactive patient is a real test of any nurse's ingenuity. She must constantly steer a middle path, meeting wherever possible, the needs of all her patients. She may gain some consolation from the fact that her patient will be easily distracted and can there-fore sometimes be channelled towards some less disrup-tive activity, and that such symptoms invariably improve with time and medication.

THE PATIENT WHO IS VIOLENT OR AGGRESSIVE

At least some of Julie's initial misgivings about psychi-atric nursing may have been due to a fear of being assaulted. Nurses during their general training frequently cite violence as being their main concern or area of uncertainity prior to this module. Perhaps they share with the general public an exaggerated misconception of the amount of violence that occurs in psychiatric hospitals.

Violent or aggressive incidents can and do take place, but nurses who spend their off duty in such activities as attending discos, football matches or pubs, or indeed, in walking down the street at night, are almost definitely in far greater danger.

In her training so far, Julie may have witnessed aggression in the accident and emergency unit, in geriatric wards or in surgical areas where perhaps sudden withdrawal may unexpectedly reveal an addiction to alcohol or drugs. These are all potential danger areas.

However, in psychiatry as elsewhere, violence when it does occur can be terrifying for the nurses and the other patients. What is less well understood is the fact that it can be even more frightening for the perpetrator. In today's society we are expected to keep a firm grip on our less desirable traits, and the feeling of losing control, even briefly, can be alarming. Nurses who may be unconsciously aware of a smouldering difficulty in controlling their own aggressive impulses are often the most punitive towards others who suddenly erupt angrily.

Reasons for violence

Management of violence can often only be effective if the events leading up to it are understood. Consequently, following each incident all precipitating factors should be carefully considered. This may prevent a recurrence.

In some, although comparatively few, cases an explanation may be directly attributable to the patient's *current symptomatology*.

Voices may urge him to lash out; he may 'see' dangerous animals that must be fought off, or he may suddenly 'realise' that a fellow patient has been sent to assassinate him. A young man with a history of impulsive behaviour may suddenly be thwarted, or an overactive, overconfident patient may be prevented from leaving the ward to negotiate a totally unrealistic business deal.

In the majority of incidents, however, there will be no such clear cut link between the patient's symptoms and his outburst. Domestic and sometimes *thoroughly understandable reasons* may be found.

The patient will be anxious on admission. Was he greeted warmly and orientated properly? He may be being nursed alongside acutely disturbed individuals. If in fact they pose no physical threat, is he aware of this? He may feel inarticulate and stupidly incompetent when it comes to verbalising his feelings in a sophisticated group setting. Was he left with no other channel for expressing his views? Other patients or staff may have abrasive personalities. Is his outburst an understandable reaction to such a person?

Very occasionally, there may be *a physical reason* such as hypoglycaemia in a diabetic, or in the periods leading up to or immediately following a convulsion in an epileptic. Premenstrually, some women are subject to dramatic mood and personality changes.

Nursing management of violence

Defusing a potentially violent episode

It is certainly true that prevention is better than cure, and while hopefully, Julie will never encounter overt violence during her module, she will meet patients who are disgruntled, or otherwise close to lashing out.

A calm, interested approach to such an individual is important. Julie can walk a little with him, or sit down and talk in a quiet corner. The source of his annoyance can possibly be dealt with; he can be encouraged to ignore an argumentative companion, or to leave the television room if the programme is not to his liking. By engaging him in table tennis or pool, Julie can help him relax, and while in this more informal atmosphere he may verbalise his emotions more easily.

As a useful but usually unnecessary precaution, it seems sensible to explain her intentions to a fellow member of staff before going with a potentially disturbed patient to an area where immediate help may not be available.

Handling overt violence

Should actual violence flare up, there may be little prior warning, and thus planning for individual incidents may be difficult. Consequently, only broad principles can be considered.

The following outcomes should be striven for:

a. The patient should be unhurt during the incident.
b. Staff should be unhurt during the incident.
c. Other patients who may be in the vicinity or who may become involved, should be unhurt.
d. Damage to property should be kept to a minimum.

Physical 'battles' should be avoided if at all possible. One-to-one confrontations are particularly unhelpful, since they may tempt the patient to think that he has a chance of 'winning' provided he is even more violent. In addition, once the incident is over it will be difficult to readjust to a normal nurse/patient relationship if the struggle can be construed as having been a personal one. A nurse hurt in a violent clash, will, over and above the discomfort she may suffer, be unable to look after the other patients in her care.

If a patient requires to be restrained, therefore, it is far better to summon help. He can then be approached *calmly and in sufficient numbers* to reduce the likelihood of injury, and to convince him that a fight will be futile. Staff should have a prearranged plan as to who will do what, thus avoiding the farcical situation of everyone diving for the same leg. The patient should be swiftly transferred to the floor where he can most readily be immobilised by firmly holding the major joints of the shoulders and hips. His boots or shoes should be removed. In this position, he is least likely to hurt himself or to inflict serious injury on others.

Although a patient cannot be restrained indefinitely the decision to release him should not be taken lightly. To allow him back on his feet immediately may precipitate further violence so a gradual letting go is preferable. The nurse in charge should talk quietly to the still immobilised patient. He may point out the staff's superior numbers and try to obtain a promise that the patient will not immediately resort to violence if he is allowed back on his feet. Perhaps surprisingly, a promise thus made is often kept.

Any violent fracas will result in the sending for a doctor, and on his arrival, a tranquillising drug may be prescribed. The ready availability of such drugs means that episodes of violence are commonly short-lived and that more physical forms of restraint are now obsolete.

Because of its comparative rarity an incident such as the one described above will be a major talking point in the ward where it occurs. The patient involved may be frightened and embarrassed, and will be totally unsure of how he will be treated from then on. It is important that the nurse in charge, both verbally and by his general attitude, makes it absolutely clear that *no victimisation* will take place. Violence cannot be condoned but it is the patient's actions — not him as a person — that are unacceptable. He must be left in no doubt that this is so.

Entirely satisfactory guidelines as to how much force can be used to quell a violent outburst do not exist. Clearly however, it must be the minimum amount necessary to achieve its aim, after giving due consideration to all the circumstances.

Coping with an old man in a psychogeriatric ward who lashes out with his stick need require no more than a

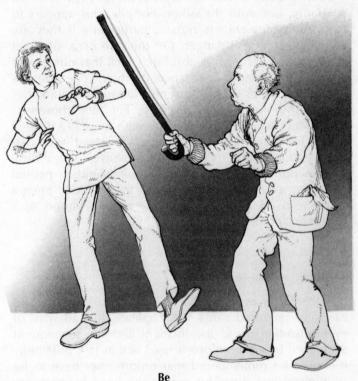

**Be
on your
guard!**

hasty leap out of his reach and a sense of humour. On the other hand, a physically fit young man intent on inflicting injury would have to be repelled with some strength.

Some groups of workers are known for their sense of *solidarity*, one with the other. Happily, this appears to exist among psychiatric nurses, particularly if they are faced with physical danger. On the rare occasions that violence does erupt it is absolutely vital that nurses can rely on the speedy assistance of their colleagues — something which they in turn must unquestionably offer should the situation be reversed. For Julie, however, such direct action is unlikely, although there is a distinct possibility that she may find herself involved in a *crisis intervention group* (Ch. 8). This involves the critical examination by everyone in the vicinity plus a neutral chairman, of events leading up to the incident. Such a group can do much to minimise the likelihood of a similar incident occurring.

Reporting violent incidents

It is absolutely essential that all episodes of violence are carefully recorded. This will facilitate the analysis of events leading up to the incident and the subsequent avoidance of a repetition. If legal action is a possibility it should be remembered that reports may have to be scrutinised in court. This makes the need for accuracy even more important.

When patients are in hospital for a prolonged period and treatment is not particularly active, there is a grave danger that the occasional aggressive outburst is almost all that will be reported. Incidents separated by considerable periods of time may thus be close to each other in the patient's file giving a false impression of their frequency. This tendency may be partly countered by reporting positive events when appropriate and by clearly dating each report of aggression.

Possibly because of their relative rarity, violent incidents tend to provide a talking point among staff. It is vitally important for both confidentiality and accuracy that anecdotes about aggressive patient's should not be exaggerated.

Once a patient has a reputation for violence, staff may unwittingly communicate to him their apprehension or readiness for conflict. This may have the totally undesirable effect of provoking further, preventable episodes.

THE PATIENT WHO IS CONFUSED

Confusion should rightly be considered a symptom rather than a specific disease. Its importance lies in its comparative commonness, its possible treatability and the demands it makes on the nurse's time.

Julie will have seen many confused patients during the course of her work in general wards and will appreciate that the symptoms can be either *acute* or *chronic* in their presentation.

Discovering the cause

Doctors and nurses must unite in trying to discover the cause of the confusional episodes. Chronic states or dementia should be diagnosed only after all treatable alternatives have been discounted.

The following are a selection of treatable causes of confusion:

Infection — the delirium sometimes seen in measles or the confusion associated with bronchopneumonia or urinary tract infection in the elderly. Encephalitis or meningitis may also be important.

Intoxication — this may involve alcohol, drugs (withdrawal as well as excess), industrial substances or (more topically) solvents.

Head injury — intracranial bleeding may be chronic with minimal bleeding from a slight injury which may be forgotten before the symptoms appear.

Cardiovascular problems — anything which inhibits an adequate supply of oxygenated blood being pumped towards the brain.

Dehydration/malnutrition

Diabetes mellitus — usually due to hypoglycaemia.

Epilepsy — particularly following a tonic/clonic seizure.

Surgery or anaesthesia

Constipation

Unfamiliar surroundings.

Principles of care

Apart from the symptomatic treatment of these causative factors, several broad principles apply when nursing the confused patient.

It should be remembered that confusion frequently gets worse during the hours of darkness, particularly in the presence of stimuli that can be easily misinterpreted. Nurses whispering to avoid disturbing their patients may be mistaken for intruders planning their misdeeds. Articles of clothing lying around may appear to be a person lurking in the darkness. Cot sides on the bed, if not recognised as such, may make the patient feel entrapped. Consequently, he may try to escape by climbing over them, perhaps precipitating the type of accident they were supposed to prevent.

Distractions should be kept to a minimum, and for this reason patients are best nursed in a *single room*. A simple night light, bright enough to illuminate dark corners but dim enough to promote relaxation, should be provided.

If *night sedation* is required, both the dose and the time of administration must be carefully calculated. A drug given too late in the night may send the patient to sleep for most of the next day, leading to his being full of life once again the following evening.

Patient-orientated care is important and the confused person should, whenever possible, be attended by the same calm, tolerant nurse. Momentary restraint, if for instance an individual who is very confused is climbing over his cot sides, should be friendly but firm, and relaxed as soon as possible.

A lot of noisy, active visitors may further confuse the patient, and if so, they must be discouraged. The presence of one familiar and quiet relative or friend, however, may exert a calming influence and should therefore be welcomed.

Chronic confusion

Despite the treatability of much confusion, some patients seem destined to remain at least partly confused. Their condition is likely to be part of the clinical picture presented by dementia, which is discussed in greater detail in Chapter 14.

A diagnosis of dementia often condemns the patient to a self-fulfilling prophecy of hopelessness as they spiral downwards towards increasing dependency. Sometimes his condition will worsen dramatically on entering hospital. At home, where everything is familiar, his tentative grip on his surroundings may be just sufficient to allow him to get by. However, he may be totally unable to assimilate the host of new information necessary to orientate him to this strange environment.

Regretably psychogeriatric wards have been seen in the past as places of no hope. Likewise their inhabitants have been designated as being on the 'scrap heap' and the care provided has been custodial and uninspired.

This is unforgivable. Cures will not be a feature of these wards, but it is undeniable that psychogeriatric patients deserve as high a standard of physical and psychological care as any other group in hospital.

In planning a personal care plan for her patients Julie will be faced with many diverse nursing problems which will encroach on environmental as well as more traditional matters.

Providing a homely atmosphere

It is difficult to make a stark Nightingale ward reminiscent of home, yet it is important to try. Imaginative use of room dividers is an excellent start, while the smaller areas thus achieved can at least in part be individually decorated. Duvet covers which can be bright and easily washed should not all be the same, nor should they be chosen to satisfy the prejudices of the staff. Floor carpets do much to create an atmosphere of cosy homeliness, but are of course less than ideal if constantly saturated with urine. However, when practical, their use should be encouraged.

Personal ornaments can do much to remind the patient who is chronically confused of home. A photograph of a grandchild or a dog will evoke happy memories, establish the patient as an unique individual, and help identify his locker or bed. Unfortunately the safety of such personal treasures cannot be guaranteed in an environment where several individuals may be muddled or unwittingly destructive. Nevertheless, while this should be pointed out to the relatives, it should not be used as an excuse to do nothing.

Reality orientation (RO)

Reality orientation is widely practised in long-term wards catering for the elderly confused since this is the group of patients who seem to derive most benefit from its application.

24-hour RO. This is more an overall philosophy than a specific treatment. Everything in the patient's environment and everybody involved in the care must be geared towards maintaining the patient's orientation. Wards should be adequately signposted, while clocks, calendars, menus and weather charts should be prominently displayed and of a size that can be read by ageing eyes. This can be more easily provided than a consistently dynamic and positive attitude in the nursing staff. Yet both are crucial

At the end of the first of a two lecture series on cerebral vascular accidents, the author recently announced that he would rejoin the class at 2.15 to finish the discussion. A student in the front row pointed out that according to the timetable the lesson was scheduled to start at 3.15. The author checked his diary, acknowledged she was right, and the incident was allowed to pass.

This anecdote is noteworthy only because it is so commonplace. During the course of our normal day-to-day functioning many of us make little slips, or forget things momentarily. Because we have not been labelled 'confused', 'demented', or maybe even just elderly, we are immediately corrected, usually gently, and so are unwittingly kept firmly in touch with reality. Frequently this corrective courtesy is not extended to the patient who is already confused.

> Mr Kelly is pleasantly confused and requires a good deal of assistance with dressing. He tends, in particular, to get muddled with the days of the week. As the nurse hurriedly dressed him, Mr Kelly announced, 'Tommorow my daughter and grandaughter will visit.'
> The nurse, a kindly person replied, 'Super, Mr Kelly! You will be looking forward to that.'
> Mr Kelly nodded contentedly.

The incident took place on a Wednesday morning and Mr Kelly's visitors invariably attend on a Sunday. So Mr Kelly had got it wrong. In fact he got it wrong most of the time, and the conversation was typical. His visitors, according to him, were usually coming 'tommorow'. It was quicker and possibly even less upsetting to agree with him, yet in so doing, the nurse was denying him the right to reorientate himself — a right which is usually given automatically to the rest of us.

Her response should have been, 'Doesn't your daughter usually visit on Sunday? This is only Wednesday, Mr Kelly. Your daughter will come in 4 days time. I'm sure you must be looking forward to it.'

It is paradoxical that those of us who are supposedly 'normal', have our mistakes rectified, while others with acknowledged difficulties are allowed to muddle through.

Class RO. This takes place in a more formal session, lasting perhaps half an hour, and is supplementary to the 24-hour RO. Here, orientation is more deliberately taught; the weather is discussed, the ward notice board may be changed, while flowers may be smelled and identified. These classes are made up of a small group of patients who, if carefully selected, may prove mutually supportive.

The nurse in her capacity as group leader has a definite responsibility to ensure that patients who have substantially deteriorated, do not have their shortcomings highlighted and are spared the embarrassment of continual mistakes.

Why RO?

One argument states that reality orientation is in fact inappropriate, and that patients in, for example, a psychogeriatric ward, are better off confused and/or disorientated and thus blissfully unaware of their hapless surroundings. This theory may seem superficially attractive. We may be able to recall the frustration of a patient who has been aware of his slow deterioration, and on comparing this with the indifference of someone more completely disorientated, we may be tempted to think that the former condition is less desirable.

This is a defeatest attitude. Although the merit in continuously reminding an old person of something, like the death of a spouse, which they specifically want to forget is dubious, to encourage blanket forgetfulness is to encourage dependence.

Independence for her patients, even though limited to seemingly insignificant areas of their life, must be the nurse's goal.

Reminiscence

Julie will almost certainly have been struck by some of her patients' ability to recall the past. Although having little or no recollection about even major happenings of a few hours ago, an elderly patient may relate with pleasure minute details concerning his schooldays.

By harnessing these memories, Julie can stimulate the old person's mind and also increase her own knowledge of a bygone era. By introducing old photographs, (most families have them somewhere) or mementoes of long past historic events such as royal weddings, she can help her patients recall their youth. Old gramophone records and newspaper clippings can similarly jolt the memory, while an ambitious dimension can be added by encouraging them to recall and subsequently cook traditional recipes. The party spirit engendered during such occasions is in stark contrast to the depressingly familiar scenes of apathy which they may have replaced.

Permanent 'living in the past' is usually discouraged as being a sign of advanced dementia, but the occasional planned trip down memory lane can be both enjoyable and therapeutic.

The nursing care of a confused patient, chronic or acute, is time consuming and not always immediately rewarding, yet it is an increasingly important part of the nurse's responsibility. At present the field in not static and changes, though unspectacular, are taking place. As with reality orientation and reminiscence, it seems likely that nurses will be in the forefront of all improvements in this important area.

THE PATIENT WHO IS INCONTINENT

Incontinence is by no means confined to the psychiatric patient, but as the proportion of elderly patients steadily increases, it claims an increasing amount of many nurse's time. Some wards have a characteristic smell of stale urine which is demoralising but very difficult to eradicate.

As elsewhere, a surprising amount of the incontinence in psychogeriatric wards can be remedied with good nursing care. Furthermore, perseverance on the part of the nurse will bring about at least some degree of improvement in almost all cases. Causes should be actively sought. Some, if discovered, may lead to remarkable progress in a short space of time. Urinary infection, oversedation or constipation are all very treatable, while some patients with urgency will improve if provided with a commode or if their bed or favourite chair is moved nearer the toilet.

It seems likely that if nurses concentrated on treating incontinence or establishing continence rather than merely cleaning, drying and changing patients after the event, they would actually reduce their workload. Furthermore, such work would surely by more pleasant, and a morale booster for both nurse and patient.

Patients must be offered toilet facilities regularly since many will be unable to ask. A written record can be kept with little extra demand on the nurse's time. However it is essential that continence and any successful use of the toilet is recorded as well as any episodes of incontinence. When such charts are kept for even a short period of time a pattern may emerge and it frequently becomes possible to anticipate when a patient is likely to pass urine.

Jock, who sits all day on a geriatric chair, normally passes urine at approximately 11.15 a.m. In wards practising task-orientated care, Jock and his fellow patients may be 'checked' and taken to the toilet at 12 noon prior to lunch. Jock would invariably be found to be wet and would require to be washed and changed by nurses who may already feel pressurised for time because of the impending meal. Fresh underpants and trousers would be required. Jock would have sat wet for at least half an hour, and because he had been incontinent the procedure would offer no opportunity for praise or positive reinforcement.

Armed with the information on the *continence chart* and unfettered by arbitary timetables the nurse responsible for Jock's individual care could arrange to take him to the toilet at say 11 a.m. when the chances are that he would be dry, and he may use the toilet appropriately. He could then be rewarded with genuine praise from the nurse, and furthermore, would avoid the discomfort of being wet or the indignity of being stripped and changed.

It is of course far too simplistic to suggest that such a regime would end all incontinence but it will almost definitely improve matters. Further improvements may occur if toilets are bright, warm and odour free; the type of place you could visit without turning your stomach. They must be kept scrupulously clean.

The universal man/woman symbols, a brightly coloured door, or arrows on the walls or floors will help concentrate the mind of the person who is mobile but slightly disorientated.

Most of all, the nurse's attitude must be such that

continence is considered the norm. Incontinence must be seen as something requiring active nursing intervention and the habit of waiting for it to occur so that the patient can then be changed, must be deplored.

Some incontinence is of course intractable. If this is so, then the nurse's role is clear. The patient must be kept clean and dry as much as possible and his dignity must be closely protected. Nurses will be aware of the problems associated with catheterisation, which should usually be avoided. An additional problem with many of this group of patients is the fact that they will not understand why the catheter has been passed and may well try to pull it out, risking urethral damage.

THE PATIENT WHO REFUSES TO EAT

This is another nursing problem which may be neither 'psychiatric' nor bizzare. In several of the previous sections of this chapter emphasis has been made on the need to ensure a proper diet. Yet a substantial minority of psychiatric patients will refuse, or be unable, to take their food. This presents the nurse with a considerable dilemma. As with horses and water, it is easy to proffer the food, but very difficult to ensure that it is eaten.

Although vital for life, eating for most people is much more than just a means of avoiding death. Most of us enjoy eating, and in many households, mealtimes are one of the few occasions when the whole family sits down together. We use specific food to mark special occasions, and we demonstrate our congeniality by sharing meals with our friends. Sometimes what we eat is governed by religious or cultural customs or taboos, while more formally, our likes, dislikes and dietary eccentricities help establish each of us as an unique individual.

The ability to refuse food wilfully is a powerful

weapon. The toddler may be amazed to discover that his previously omnipotent mother can do little if he declines a meal. Overreaction from parents at this point may sow the seeds for prolonged battles of will over the dining room table, when instead, they should bear in mind, that a healthy, hungry toddler will not allow himself to starve.

Self starvation as a means of furthering a cause is an ancient but powerful ploy. This century the strength of emotion engendered by *Mahatma Gandhi*, and more recently, political *hunger strikers*, adequately demonstrates the exalted importance we attach to the consumption of food.

Psychiatric patients may refuse to eat for many reasons. They may feel that they are unworthy of food or that they cannot afford to pay for it. They may be so busy that they have no time for such mundane activities, or may be prevented from getting started by the need to carry out time-consuming rituals. They may be too confused to recognise food or to know what to do with it. Suspicious patients may feel that their food is being poisoned, while refusal to eat is the predominant symptom of *anorexia nervosa* and the establishment of a more 'normal' attitude to food is a major goal in its treatment.

When faced with such intransigence, two points are worth making. Firstly, the patient's mental condition may require urgent treatment from the medical staff, e.g. an overactive individual may require a tranquillising drug. Secondly, it should be made plain that a patient will not be allowed to die and will if necessary be artificially fed. This of course would involve the nurse and may raise certain ethical questions.

In practice, however, not all cases of food refusal are the result of a serious psychiatric complaint. When food is left untouched, the nurse must resist the temptation to attribute it automatically to the patient's mental condition.

Thank goodness for Julie! Non-psychiatrically-orientated nurses, perhaps unwittingly, may spot the more *straightforward explanations* and their response, based on commonsense rather than obscure psychological reasoning, may be just what's required.

Does he have proper fitting dentures? she may wonder. Are they in position? Is the food palatable and at the right temperature? His dietary preferences will be noted in his nursing history. Are they being considered? Is the food served attractively? Are the surroundings congenial?

It is not easy to cater for the large number of individuals who inhabit institutions such as our psychiatric hospitals. Catering staff adequately meet the nutritional needs of our patients and are usually skilled at providing *special diets*, whether it be for medical or religious reasons. They cannot, however, be expected to attend to the individual preferences of every patient. The nurse, on the other hand, must try to do just that!

Some patients will like their tea strong, others must have it weak. Some only like coffee, while others never drink beverages at all. Small tables for four or six people allow individuals with similar preferences to sit together in a more 'normal' atmosphere and are vastly preferable to rows of institutional furniture.

Meals, attractively presented, served at the correct temperature, on crack-free crockery will encourage patients to eat. It is better to offer second helpings later than to overfill the plates of possibly reluctant eaters.

Most patients have at least some money to spend on themselves and may elect to buy a jar of instant coffee or a pack of biscuits — such freedom of choice is desirable. Many people enjoy an occasional 'carry out' from an Indian or Chinese restaurant and a group of patients may likewise wish to indulge themselves. This should be seen as a welcome expression of their individuality rather than a criticism of hospital food.

Some patients will require painstaking feeding, some will have to be encouraged or cajoled before they eat anything; Julie already has the skills to handle this. Others may have disgusting or antisocial eating habits. In order to preserve the dignity of these individuals and to provide the majority with a more acceptable environment, they should eat by themselves, under the close supervision of a nurse. In such circumstances, reintegration with the rest of the patients in the main dining area may represent a worthwhile treatment goal.

THE PATIENT WHO IS INSTITUTIONALISED

A large number of patients who have been in hospital for other than a short stay will show signs of institutionalisation. Since most long-term psychiatric patients have a diagnosis of schizophrenia, they more than any other group, are likely to suffer from superimposed institutionalisation. As a result, the condition was not immediately recognised; the symptoms were attributed instead to the inevitable result of schizophrenia.

It is now unclear whether it is schizophrenia or its 'treatment' that is primarily responsible for the pathetic specimens of humanity, for so long a feature of our back wards. It seems likely to be the latter.

Barton (1959) in his still relevant publication *Institutional Neurosis* summarised the condition as being a disease characterised by apathy, lack of initiative, loss of interest (especially of things of an impersonal nature), submissiveness, apparent inability to make plans for the future, lack of individuality and sometimes a characteristic gait.

Julie, will on her first day on the ward, instantly recognise patients who fit this description. Perhaps they will be sitting staring into space or pacing aimlessly accross the floor or hospital grounds. They may, in all weathers, run trivial messages for staff, who may be two generations their junior.

Goffman (1961) spoke of *total institutions* and discovered similarities in them all. Military camps, prisoner of war camps, sanatoria, prisons, some religious orders and remote places of work such as logging camps, he classed as total institutions. In contrast to 'normal' life, inmates tended to eat, sleep and spend their free time in the company of the same 'batch' of companions, in a time-tabled existence, geared very much to the needs of the institution. Traditional mental hospitals, built well out in the country and largely self-sufficient fitted smoothly into this pattern. Staff accommodation was provided and many members of the same family tended to live, work and get a good deal of their recreation within the hospital walls. It is hardly surprising that such members of staff became rather inward-looking and tended to cut themselves off from the outside world. If this can happen to the workers, the outlook for patients is grim indeed!

Young nurses like Julie, professionally naive, but full of bright ideas and dedicated to the dignity of man, unwittingly play a major role in counterbalancing this trend. A fresh face, just passing through, serves as a reminder that out there is a whole big world. Fresh ideas, although in shorter supply, are the main weapon in the battle against institutionalisation. Administrative expediency has long meant that individual's likes, dislikes and eccentricities are largely ignored as they carry out their limited daily activities as one of a large group.

Yet in some instances, a planned, positive rehabilitative effort can reverse the ravages of institutionalisation. For example, patients who may have been mute, and/or incontinent can again develop much more socially acceptable habits.

The benefits of planned care have been described in Chapter 2. In an effort to meet individual needs, assessment of the patient's problems, both actual and potential, is of course essential. Too often, it is still considered highly innovative. Equally important, is the allocating of a nurse or nurses who will be primarily responsible for each patient's care, including the close liaison between a wide variety of carers from other disciplines. Consistency of approach is vital.

Care planning for the most institutionalised patients must be very basic. Before anything else, they must relearn to wash, groom and keep themselves clean, use the toilet appropriately and conduct themselves in a reasonable manner at the table. Paradoxically, this may first be achieved in *small groups*. Unlike Goffman's 'batches', however, these groups will be carefully selected. They will be small, consist of patients with similar problems and objectives and will be mainly under the direct guidance of 'their' own nurse or nurses.

Initially, it may be necessary to adhere strictly to time-tables so that one small group dovetails with another and fits into the overall ward plan. Nevertheless, the totally unforgivable sight of large queues of patients hanging around in various stages of undress, waiting to use inadequate toilet facilities, in conditions which are far from private, should be eradicated.

As the nurse cajoles and encourages ('reinforces' in the language of behaviour therapists) her patients towards greater achievements, she must beware. Such a directive approach while necessary at the start must be dropped as soon as possible in favour of a more democratic regime. Otherwise dependence and continued institutionalisation will be encouraged.

It is often said that once patients have been in hospital for perhaps 2 years, their families will have become used to life without them. Reintegration into the community after such a period of time can therefore be difficult. While nowadays this is recognised and great emphasis is placed on early discharge, even although subsequent readmission is likely to be necessary, there are still patients who have been in our hospitals for many years.

When applicable, contact should be re-established with family or former friends. This is usually seen as being one of the roles of the social worker, but the original suggestion may well come from an enthusiastic nurse. The nurse can help her patient with the first, faltering letter, and may later accompany him on what may be a difficult visit.

At another level, two-way communication with the community should be maintained. Concert parties, lecturers, soccer teams and youth groups can be encouraged to visit. Patients may go (accompanied at first, but later, if all goes well, on their own) to their church, a soccer match, for a pub lunch or to whatever they fancy. This to-ing and fro-ing helps remind the patient of life outside the constraints of hospital, and equally importantly, helps educate the public on mental illhealth.

Throughout this book we emphasise the need for a humane and empathic nursing approach, and rightly or wrongly, tacitly assume that such attitudes are inherent in most nurses. Sadly, there are exceptions.

Teasing, *bullying* or *bossiness* by 'rogue' members of staff can result in apathy and withdrawal on the part of the patients. Such staff attitudes must be eradicated, either by encouragement and counselling, or as a last resort, by disciplinary or legistlative action.

The effect of medication

The contribution of *chemotherapy* to modern psychiatry should not be minimised. However, drugs overprescribed and inadequately reviewed, play a major part in producing the so-called 'zombies' in long-term care. When major tranquillisers are withdrawn by the doctor, the patient may immediately show more spontaneity and interest. Florid psychiatric symptoms may not return, but if they do, they may well be controlled by a greatly reduced dosage.

Patients should be constantly reminded of the prospect of life outside hospital and we shall see in Chapter 4 how a gradual reintroduction to the community is, with support, sometimes possible. The task of placing an ex-psychiatric patient in open competitive employment has never been easy, and with the current trend away from 'jobs for all', it will become increasingly difficult. However, some will be lucky, and for others, living an independent life in accommodation outside the hospital, may be an acceptable compromise.

Before this stage can be reached, the atmosphere and administration of the ward itself may require close scrutiny. A friendly, homely atmosphere should be actively promoted and each patient should have at least some private space around his bed, in the shape of a wardrobe, chest of drawers or such like.

> Charlie had been in hospital for 65 of his 70 odd years, and puzzled staff with his magpie type behaviour. All manner of useless trivia was hoarded by Charlie and stuffed under his mattress, in the lining of his jacket or in his ever present cap. Yet was his behaviour so unusual?

Many nurses, I am sure, would cringe at the prospect of having the contents of their handbags, pockets or dressing table drawers exposed to scrutiny. Most of us seem to collect useless bits and pieces along the way. Their significance, if remembered, is important only to us, and all that they have in common is that they are *personal*.

Charlie has been well-fed and kept in increasing comfort over the years, but has had little opportunity to amass life's trinkets. That he tries, even inappropriately, to do so should be applauded.

Charlie should not have to hide away his treasures surreptitiously. Personal belongings must be encouraged as a means of expressing individuality, and space is required to display them.

In some instances the whole culture of the ward is deliberately changed and a more democratic regime is introduced. Patients are encouraged to play an active part in the day-to-day running of the ward and may find themselves making decisions for the first time in years.

Chapter 8 deals more fully with the therapeutic community and looks in greater detail at the exciting attempts at de-institutionalisation and giving back to the patients at least some responsibility for the running of their own lives.

WHAT NOW FOR JULIE?

The above chapter looked at several problems common in, but not exclusive to, psychiatric nursing. Hopefully, Julie will be relieved to find some things that are familiar, and perhaps now, she can more confidently tackle those that are not.

In the pages that follow, in which we examine in closer detail features specific to psychiatric nursing and psychiatry, we leave Julie temporarily behind. But it is for all the 'Julies' in nursing that this book is written.

REFERENCES

Barton R 1959 Institutional neurosis. Wright, Bristol
Goffman E 1961 Asylums: Essays on the social situation of mental
    patients and other inmates. Penguin, Harmondsworth
Wells T J 1980 Problems in geriatric nursing care. Churchill
    Livingstone, Edinburgh

The Community Psychiatric Nurse (CPN)
Functions of the CPN
The development of the CPN
Community facilities for the
   psychiatrically disordered

4

Psychiatric community care

In recent decades there has been a definite move away from the concept of the large institution. Its role in the care of the psychiatrically disordered is now openly questioned.

As society becomes more accepting and the horrors of long-term institutionalisation are fully appreciated, the idea of community care is increasingly attractive. In any shift of emphasis away from psychiatric hospitals, the part played by the *Community Psychiatric Nurse* (CPN) is obviously important.

THE COMMUNITY PSYCHIATRIC NURSE

In 1954, two nurses were seconded from Warlingham Park Hospital to Croydon Borough to care for discharged psychiatric patients in the community. This is generally considered to have heralded the dawn of community psychiatric nursing and came about for two main reasons:

   (i) an increased awareness of the desirability of the

      continued supervision of many patients following discharge

(ii) a shortage of psychiatric social workers.

In 1957, Moorhaven Hospital started its community psychiatric service for similar reasons, but its nurses remained attached to the hospital, carrying out the dual role of community/hospital nurses.

Both these examples were extensively copied and even today, there is no real agreement as to whether the CPN should best be based in the hospital or perhaps in a Health Centre.

Being hospital-based means that CPNs have a greater opportunity of getting to know new patients prior to their discharge and vice versa. They are likely to have more ready access to ward meetings and case presentations and closer contact with the psychiatrists and hospital-based team.

On the other hand, attachment to a health centre emphasises the nurse's community role, counteracting the tendency to associate psychiatric disorder inevitably with hospitalisation. They are more likely to be accepted on an equal footing by other primary care workers. This may lead to more rapid communication and a reduction of costly overlaps in function.

This basic uncertainty perhaps arose because of the fact that community psychiatric nursing services sprang up in piecemeal fashion, largely as a result of locally felt needs. Initially there was no national policy and CPNs probably performed very different functions.

Perhaps there is something to be said for a system which has been tailored towards the real life situation and these administrative inconsistencies may not be important.

Functions of the Community Psychiatric Nurse

Supervision of drug therapy

As we have seen, the earliest CPNs were involved solely in follow-up work with ex-psychiatric patients. This seemed sensible as discharge from hospital can be a threatening experience with readmission always a worrying possibility.

Historically, many patients of long standing were able to leave hospital following the introduction of the *major tranquillising drugs* in the 1950s.

However, some unforeseen problems arose.

Re-establishing community links is not easy. Many changes will have taken place and family, if still around, may not necessarily be welcoming. In addition, patients who might have been prescribed a combination of drugs to be taken as often as four times daily, almost invariably stopped taking them. Relapses became inevitable.

These problems were greatly reduced by the introduction of long acting phenothiazines, such as Modecate (fluphenazine decanoate) which could be given intramuscularly at intervals of between 2 and 4 weeks. Each patient could call at a 'Modecate clinic' in the hospital or health centre at these relatively infrequent intervals, or a community nurse could visit them at home.

These drugs meant that it was much easier to check that patients were getting their tranquillisers, while the regular contact ensured they would be monitored for side-effects or relapses. Psychological or practical support was frequently sought and given along with the injection, and the need for further nursing involvement could be assessed.

Mr R. (42 years old) lives with his elderly mother and works in a piggery. After almost 7 years in a psychiatric hospital he was discharged on Modecate 4 years ago. He leads a solitary but contented life and just having him at home after all those years is a source of great comfort to his mother. The

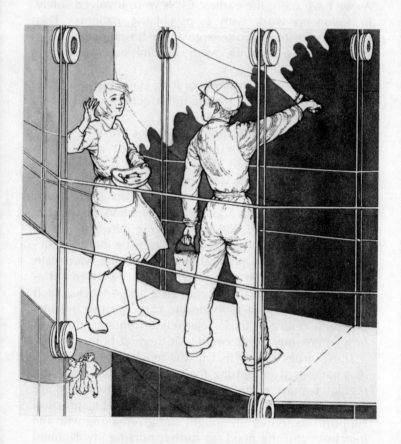

Treating the patient in the community

CPN visits once every 3 weeks to give him his injection and although her contact lasts for less than 15 minutes it is enjoyed by all. It is an important event in Mr R.'s life.

This giving of long-acting phenothiazines and the close monitoring of those receiving them is an important part of the CPN's work.

Other ex-patients, particularly those on lithium salts or the type of anti-depressants known as monoamine oxidase inhibitors, (MAOIs) may require regular visits when any side-effects can be noted.

The patient and his family

Although still at school, Margo's continual refusal to eat had come close to killing her, causing serious problems for her parents and elder sister. At one stage these had almost caused the complete breakdown of the family.

During 3 months in hospital, Margo regained her 'target' weight, and the whole family had a chance to look at themselves more closely in therapy sessions with a psychiatrist and psychiatric nurse.

As her discharge date loomed ever closer, the CPN became increasingly involved.

Now that Margo has been discharged, the CPN visits once a fortnight, seeing the whole family together. These visits last much longer than the time spent with Mr R., and are psychologically more taxing, but they are crucial to the family's well-being and continued existence.

On still other occasions the CPN may adopt the role of individual rather than family therapist, perhaps working closely with her patient on a systematic desensitisation or other clearly defined programme.

The CPN as an alternative to hospital admission

Wayne (19 years old) lived in an area where unemployment was chronically very high, but unlike most of his former schoolmates he had a reasonably paid job in a garage.

From time to time, Wayne would become extremely over anxious, agitated and unable to concentrate. At such times, he required professional help but his GP had become increasingly aware of his own lack of success in treating him.

At present, Wayne attends a psychiatrist as an outpatient once a month, but may be seen as often as twice weekly by the CPN. So far he has avoided the need for hospitalisation and therefore the stigma of being labelled a patient. Most importantly, his work suffers only minor disruptions and he remains in employment.

Psychiatric hospitalisation is always a major event for the person concerned. It should not be suggested unless it seems likely that its attendant disadvantages will be outweighed by its benefits. Normally it should be offered only when less drastic measures seem doomed to fail.

Individuals who are frightened of losing their job, who have a young family at home to look after, or who are frightened by the myths of what goes on in mental hospitals may with justification refuse admission. The CPN may be a suitable alternative in providing the care which they require and to which they are entitled.

Crisis intervention

Life is full of unexpected events which may temporarily throw us and test our ability to cope. For some, this ability may be found wanting. Ex-psychiatric patients, their families and others who may have a psychological disturbance may get by adequately most of the time, as long as they know that someone will be there should things go badly wrong.

The CPN may well be that someone and her response to this cry for help is known as crisis intervention.

A daughter caring for a dementing father may be temporarily overwhelmed when he floods the bathroom. An alcoholic who restarts drinking may threaten the stability of his family, or an adolescent may strike out at his mother. These are crises.

To be effective, crisis intervention should occur

immediately and when successful, will lead to a reappraisal of the home circumstances and a better understanding of how things may be handled in the future.

On occasions direct action may be necessary. The old man may have reached the stage when he must be admitted to hospital but this is not the aim of crisis intervention. The knowledge that professional help is only a phone call away is comforting. It can be the difference between a family staying intact and working through its difficulties, or having one of its members singled out as a patient, and being sent to hospital.

The CPN on this type of visit must beware of taking sides, either for or against her 'patient', and when necessary should temper her support with a tactful interpretation of the dynamics of the situation.

Education and prevention

In many ways the CPNs are in the frontline in the battle against psychiatric disorder. They are most likely to come into contact with GPs, health visitors and district nurses, who in turn, may be in a position to recognise potential psychological problems before they become a crisis. They may have personal contacts with police, teachers, the clergy or community leaders. Through discussion and by example, the CPNs may establish themselves as the legitimate link with the more traditional psychiatric services. In areas where a high percentage of the population belongs to an ethnic minority group it would be ideal if the CPN came from a similar background. If not she must familiarise herself completely with the dominant customs and norms of the culture.

More formally, the CPN may have the opportunity to meet with and address various local organisations and community groups. This educating role should be welcomed as an important part of the struggle to demystify psychiatric disorder.

The development of the CPN

The community psychiatric nursing service has come a long way in a comparatively short time. Although general nurse learners will not spend long with the CPN they may be able to accompany her on a visit or two. Almost certainly, they will become increasingly aware of the importance of her work.

CPNs still have developmental problems, and areas where their role appears to overlap with others, particularly it seems, with social workers. Some continue to spend a great deal of time attending meetings within the hospital, while others may have difficulty in slotting into the hospital-based hierarchy. Nevertheless, what started as a hotch potch of local schemes has made considerable strides forward. Post-basic training, though not yet mandatory, is available in one of several approved courses and their own professional organisation, the *Community Psychiatric Nurses Association*, is in existence.

Along with the facilities described below, the CPN is directly responsible for the deinstitutionalisation of many psychiatric patients previously considered to be chronically ill.

COMMUNITY FACILITIES FOR THE PSYCHIATRICALLY DISORDERED

These facilities are mainly used by ex-patients who are gradually readjusting to life outside hospital, but may be available as an alternative to hospitalisation in some cases. As discussed elsewhere in this book, every person is so much an individual, that no single sequence of events is applicable to all. Rather, some of the following may be offered as part of a personally planned rehabilitative programme.

Day hospitals

Some patients may no longer require to be hospitalised. They may have a home to go to and possibly a family to care for them. However, they may still require a degree of supervision, perhaps because their family may not be around during the day, or because they feel they cannot cope without some relief. Patients may attend the day hospital from 1 to 5 days weekly. Besides having a midday meal they will be offered most of the facilities normally available in hospital. Day hospitals are staffed by trained psychiatric nurses with a psychiatrist and other team members on hand.

For some, day care will be brief, prior to a complete discharge, while others will attend on a long-term basis.

Day centres

Serve a similiar purpose but are not medically orientated. They are not part of the NHS and staff are not trained doctors or nurses.

Half way house

For many long-term patients, leaving hospital will be conditional on finding suitable accommodation. After many years in hospital this will not be easy.

As the name applies, a half way house serves as an intermediate step between hospital proper and so-called normal housing. They offer hostel type accommodation with a trained member of staff on hand to help supervise the taking of medicines and the ironing out of domestic problems. If the ex-patients are lucky enough to be in employment, they will leave the halfway house every morning, returning in the evening for their meal, bed and breakfast. More traditional hostels run by voluntary organisations, local authorities or private individuals will exist in some areas, but here, the trained supervision available will vary considerably.

Group homes

Many ex-psychiatric patients have adapted to living together in normal housing in the community with minimal supervision. These houses, known as group homes, may belong to the hospital and be situated close by, or may be rented from the local authority in an estate some distance away. Whether in employment or in receipt of social security payments, the occupants will meet their financial commitments like any other member of society. They seem to gain strength from the company of others in the same situation and may rally round with support if one of their number threatens a relapse.

Ex-patients social clubs

These may provide the only social activity for some shy or withdrawn ex-patients. They may be run by a voluntary organisation, but normally ex-patients are heavily involved in the administration themselves. Relatives or hospital staff may also attend.

Sheltered workshop

When an ex-patient is unable to compete in the open market for employment (and this is becoming increasingly difficult), he may benefit from attending a sheltered workshop.

Here, factory type work and conditions prevail, although trained psychiatric support is also on hand. Hopefully the individual will re-learn the work habit, get used to earning some money as a direct result of his endeavours and eventually progress to a proper job.

In times of economic boom, sheltered workshops can be reasonably successful. Unfortunately, they tend to rely on the goodwill of local companies for the awarding of contracts and during recessions, these may not be forthcoming.

It is a sad truth that many ex-long-term psychiatric patients cannot compete, physically or mentally in an open struggle for jobs. If the economic trend continues away from full employment, grave doubts must be cast on the future rehabilitative success of sheltered workshops.

Conclusion

Although the move towards discharging large numbers of psychiatric patients from hospital is to be applauded, we must learn from recent experiences in Italy and some parts of the USA. Such policies can only be successful if sufficient back-up is available in the community.

The plight of some ex-patients, socially inadequate and either living in low class lodging houses, or sleeping rough on park benches or under railway bridges, is periodically brought to our attention. Discharging patients to these conditions is certainly not progress, and is totally unacceptable.

The fact that it still occasionally happens strengthens the argument in favour of a continued expansion of community facilities.

SUGGESTED READING

Carr P J, Butterworth C A, Hodges B E 1980 Community psychiatric nursing. Churchill Livingstone, Edinburgh

Psychiatrist
Psychologist
Social worker
Occupational therapist
Diversional therapist
Social/recreational therapist
Clergyman

5

The multi-disciplinary team

Imagine the scene: A consultant surgeon is busy in theatre. He is surrounded by his specialised staff and high technology equipment. The lights are shining brightly. He is performing a cholecystectomy in his usual manner and is just about to remove the gall bladder.

Suddenly, Hazel, a young first-year nurse, leans over and taps him on the shoulder, 'Don't you think, Bertie, you should hold the whatsit in your other hand? I'm sure that's a better way of doing it!'

In such circumstances, the nurse would be guilty of a serious breach of professional etiquette. Many surgeons would not like to be loudly addressed as Bertie by a student nurse. By thumping him on the back she showed total ignorance of the all important concept of sterility, and considerable over-familiarity. Because of her lack of experience and limited training she is unlikely to know of a better way of removing gall bladders. Consequently, her suggestions will be neither sought, nor welcome.

Psychiatry, like theatre work, depends for its success on a smoothly operating team but there the similarity ends.

The psychiatrist is less of a god-like figure. When a

multidisciplinary approach is favoured, the spotlight will not necessarily always fall on him. Some psychiatrists may think it therapeutically beneficial for patients and staff to use first names, while many believe in giving to the patient a considerable say in decisions affecting his health. Better trained and more experienced he will certainly be, but he does not have a monopoly of common sense. Patients, learners and non-professional workers may all on occasion be capable of forming valuable insights and consequently, their views are usually taken seriously.

In theatre, the surgeon performs operations. The anaesthetist renders the patient unconscious and is responsible for maintaining him in an optimal physical condition. The 'scrub nurse' is responsible for handing the proper equipment to the surgeon while others will do the fetching and carrying. Opportunities during an operation for an individual to do another's job are strictly limited.

In psychiatry, the reverse is true. Particularly with the development of the therapeutic community, a definite blurring of staff roles has occurred. However, it is true that each discipline has its own area of competence and these will now be discussed.

THE MULTIDISCIPLINARY TEAM

The psychiatrist

The psychiatrist is a fully trained doctor who has chosen as his speciality, the treatment of the mentally disordered. Traditionally, he is seen as the leader of the therapeutic team and at one time enjoyed unfettered authority on a wide range of matters, many of which were totally unconnected with patient care. Although this power has largely been eroded, with, for instance, matters relating to nursing being the sole responsibility of nurse managers, overall clinical policies will be governed largely by his philosophy.

Psychiatrists may be *analytical* in orientation, believing that the individual's problems can be explained and alleviated by exploring his past in minute detail. Conversely, they may be *behaviourist*, believing that symptoms are due merely to faulty learning. The relief of symptoms rather than any complicated explanation is their aim and they attempt to achieve it by encouraging the patient to re-learn more adaptive responses.

They may favour individual psychotherapy, group psychotherapy or a therapeutic community approach. Only they and other qualified doctors are legally permitted to prescribe drugs or carry out physical treatments such as ECT.

The psychologist

The psychologist, or more accurately the clinical psychologist, possesses a university Master's degree in psychology, the study of the mind. He introduces a more scientific approach, concentrating on scores, tests and statistics as opposed to the subjective opinion of other team members.

Some of us may have entered nursing on the strength of passing an entrance examination, which we probably knew as an 'intelligence' test. During training, on courses, or when applying for jobs we may have had to compile personality questionnaires or be screened for the amount of extroversion or introversion we exhibit. It is a sobering thought that such tests usually have built-in lie detecting questions, so that our basic honesty is also scored.

The whole concept of measuring intelligence is controversial and some would say of limited benefit, but the value of such tests is in their relative ease of application and the lack of opportunity for tester bias. Patients may show previously unrecognised aspects of their character when narrating what is happening in a series of pictures they are shown, or when commenting on the famous Rorschach ink blot test.

These are known as *projective tests* and much can be inferred about how the patient currently views life by their interpretation. The psychologist's expertise and familiarity with these and other tests may be invaluable in helping formulate a diagnosis or perhaps more importantly, in developing an individual care plan.

Clinical psychologists also have a role to play in treatment. They may have specific knowledge and experience which equips them to conduct individual or group psychotherapy, and will have a major role to play in behaviour therapies such as systematic desensitisation with phobic patients. Token economy wards where institutionalised or mentally handicapped patients may be rehabilitated by a consistent system of rewards are likely to be planned by a clinical psychologist who will be closely involved in their administration and in teaching their principles to others, including the nursing staff.

This teaching function is an important one. Clinical psychologists are the experts on normal psychological development and consequently are well qualified to spot the abnormal. This and their special familiarity with the treatments mentioned above means they have a lot to contribute to the ongoing education of the team. Nurses should take full advantage of such learning experiences.

The treatment of the psychiatrically disordered is an imprecise science. There is a tendency to use certain treatments or approaches because they seem to work, even although their efficacy has not been completely validated. Well-established theories may have little hard evidence to back them up and cynics can have a field day ridiculing philosophies which have a widespread following.

Many psychologists have a 'feel' for research and seem not to be intimidated by the statistical jargon which can frighten nurses and some of their colleagues in other disciplines.

For the sake of our professional standing but more importantly, for the well-being of our patients, scientific research is absolutely vital. The clinical psychologist has a major role to play in any such project.

Social worker

In Chapter 4, we mentioned the similarity between the roles of the community nurse and the social worker. Although such comparisons are valid, the degree of overlap should not be exaggerated. The social worker, too, has considerable training and expertise which makes her contribution to the team different from all others.

Traditionally her role dates back many years to the time when alms were commonly distributed to the poor. Unfortunately, some people still have unrealistic ideas about the social worker's ability to pick up the bill if financial difficulties befall. The oft repeated anecdote about Mrs Smith entering the psychiatric hospital so that she 'can get her debts paid' is a gross oversimplification and largely a myth. However, many patients, and in particular the older ones, can be heard to describe the social worker as the 'welfare lady' or even the 'hospital almoner'. This sadly demonstrates a lack of knowledge regarding the wide nature of the social worker's responsibilities and may unwittingly deter those in need from asking for the help they are entitled to.

Nevertheless, the social worker is the expert in such thorny areas as the claiming of state benefits, and she should ensure that all entitlements are received and help with the filling in of official forms and documents. The mistake is in thinking that this is all she does.

A major feature of the social worker's training is its emphasis on the individual as a member of a family group or of wider society. This perhaps makes her approach less blinkered and often means that she is best equipped to deal with patients whose problems are overtly family-orientated or who are in conflict with their environment. She may be particularly sensitive to the difficulties experienced by members of *ethnic minority groups* and the implications this has on their mental well-being.

Like the community psychiatric nurse, the social worker has an important rehabilitative role to play and will follow ex-patients into the community to help them work through the difficulty of re-integration. The fact that they do not give injections or concentrate unduly on matters relating to medication, may be to their advantage. It seems possible that this allows the ex-patient to associate them with health whereas they tend to think of the nurse as being primarily involved with sickness.

The social worker has an important pivotal role to play regarding community services. She will best know what is available in any particular area and who the contact person is. She should be able to advise ex-patients and their families of facilities from which they might benefit, and can arrange for them to be offered.

The social worker also has several *legal responsibilities* and will frequently be asked by the courts for social reports on individuals who may or may not be offenders. She will be involved in the admission of some compulsory patients, while more recently she will have had a part to play in the 'second opinion' stage when patients refuse to consent to certain named treatments.

The social worker can legitimately be seen as a champion of her patients' rights. Unfortunately, she can be much maligned by the ill-informed in the community who charge her with pursuing the 'soft option' on behalf of her clients who may have broken the law. She may be caricatured as being 'Leftish', unconventional and too 'middle class' to represent ideally those in her care. Clearly, such attributes will fit some social workers, but they are too sweeping to be applied to all.

The social worker is usually skilled in interview techniques and group dynamics and plays a valuable part in multidisciplinary meetings. Her overall contribution is complicated but vital.

Occupational therapist (OT)

In the unlikely event of her wanting to offend an occupational therapist, the nurse need do no more than mention green overalls and basket weaving! As a profession, occupational therapists seem hell bent on ridding themselves of this image from the past. And this is only right because of the great change in occupational therapy over recent years.

In many psychiatric hospitals of the past, occupational therapy may have been used as a method of taking the patient's mind off his problem by giving him something to do. This rather sophisticated 'head in the sand' technique may work for ostriches but is only of limited value for many psychiatrically disturbed human beings. When all that is required is some light relief, this can become the responsibility of the diversional therapist, who lacks the specialist training of the occupational therapist.

The role of the OT in rehabilitation

The OT is a crucial member of the rehabilitative team and will be closely involved in the protracted but often successful process of re-establishing ex-psychiatric patients in the community.

As in other hospitals the OT department will include a fully functional kitchen in which the patient may re-learn, or acquire for the first time, the basic skills of preparing a meal. The occupational therapist is skilled in assessing the need for various home adaptions, or for practical aids which may assist the individual's chance of survival outwith the hospital confines. Home visits, either alone or accompanied by another member of the team, are therefore an important part of her role.

The role of the OT in acute areas

Here the biggest change has occurred. Thankfully, the spectre of whole wards of patients, shuffling often reluctantly, to the OT department in some far flung corner of the hospital is disappearing.

The haphazard and arbitrary allocation of tasks once patients have arrived there is likewise becoming a thing of the past. Planned therapy, based on their carefully assessed needs and focusing on some specific area of malfunctioning, may be beneficial. More traditional crafts may have a place in raising the self-esteem.

Projective techniques, reminiscent of the ink blot tests, are increasingly employed. This involves the patient in painting, music or pottery and then discussing in a group, the feelings their contributions arouse within them. Such therapies encourage verbalisation and insight and may be particularly invaluable for some withdrawn or inarticulate patients. An ability to draw nice pictures or play music is irrelevant, although the lack of it is frequently cited as a reason for non-participation.

Occupational therapy and the nurse

The nurse may be closer in background and function to the occupational therapist than to most other team members. This and the fact that the patient traditionally left the ward to take part in OT sometimes led to unconscious rivalry between the two disciplines. Fortunately, as the OT has become increasingly involved at ward level and participates in multidisciplinary meetings, this rivalry has less opportunity to fester. Should it still arise, it would be talked through at ward meetings.

Periodically, the nurse will be faced with disgruntled patients who refuse to attend OT, claiming that it is boring, belittling or simply a waste of time. While this may be based on fact, clearly it may also be an exaggeration or a distortion. The mechanism of *displacement* may be being used, with the aggressive feelings, which should more appropriately be voiced elsewhere, being channelled towards the comparatively safe and neutral medium of OT.

If OT is planned in a meaningful manner and specifically presented as being an important part of the treatment, and if nursing staff are consistently enthusiastic, the problem of the reluctant patient will be minimised.

Other members of the multidisciplinary team

Art, music and pottery were discussed above. Although the OT may work with all these mediums, the fortunate hospital may be able to employ specialist therapists who are highly trained in one particular area.

The **diversional therapist** who may provide games or light relief is a valued member of many teams and may be a paid employee or a volunteer.

Social/recreational therapists, who in many cases are trained psychiatric nurses with appropriate additional experience, have an increasingly important part to play in maintaining the quality of hospital life, especially for the long-term patient.

The **clergyman**, whether he be the hospital chaplain or a representative of a church in the community, will have a significant contribution to make for a considerable number of patients.

Of course the list goes on and although many members will have functions that are similar (all for instance may participate in certain groups or ward meetings) each will have his own contribution to make.

As we shall see this multidisciplinary approach can go much further. Proponents of the therapeutic community (Ch. 8) believe that everyone involved with patients, including ward domestics, tradesmen and gardeners, has something positive to offer, and more importantly, that the patients, too, have a great potential for helping each other.

For the nurse, working as a member of such a wide ranging team may be strange at first, but as her confidence grows, she is likely to find it both challenging and rewarding. Certainly it is different.

PART | # TWO

CURRENT
TREATMENT
APPROACHES

6

Physically-orientated treatment

Despite the fact that it somehow seems more sensible to treat psychological conditions by psychological means, physical treatments form a vital part of psychiatric care. Such treatments have aroused strong feelings but nevertheless, it is a fact that some of them are now established as important therapies which have helped revolutionize psychiatry.

ELECTROCONVULSIVE THERAPY (ECT)

For over 50 years, it has been accepted practice to treat various forms of psychiatric illnesses by inducing convulsions in the patients. Nowadays, electroconvulsive therapy (ECT) is the method invariably used to achieve this.

Convulsive therapy was first used by a Hungarian doctor, Von Meduna, as a result of an entirely discredited hypothesis. Because he observed that none of his schizophrenic patients seemed to suffer from epilepsy, and similarly, none of his epileptics were schizophrenic, he reasoned that the two conditions were incompatible.

He went on to postulate that by inducing epilepsy in a previously non-epileptic patient, he would cure him of schizophrenia.

Originally the convulsions were brought about by the use of drugs, such as the intramuscular injection of camphor, in oil, or later, pentamethylene-tetrazol, intravenously. Both methods were unreliable and terrifying for the patient.

In 1937, an Italian professor, Ugo Cerletti, along with his compatriot, Bini, first used electricity to produce convulsions, and ECT was born. It quickly proved more efficient than the other methods, which it largely superseded.

The original hypothesis was entirely inaccurate. It is perfectly possible for schizophrenia and epilepsy to co-exist in the same person as many psychiatric nurses can testify, but surprisingly, some of the patients showed a remarkable improvement.

Eventually it became clear that it was the depressive elements, in some schizophrenics which responded most favourably, and over the years, this has led to the use of ECT being increasingly confined to depressive illnesses, and its fall from favour elsewhere. Apart from rare instances of catatonic stupor, it seems largely ineffective in schizophrenia.

Originally given 'straight' that is without anaesthesia or muscle relaxants, ECT was a terrifying procedure for patients and staff alike, fraught with complications. These ranged from fairly minor incidents of broken teeth and bitten tongues, through a variety of muscular aches and pains, to the occasional serious occurrence of broken limbs and crushed vertebrae. Mercifully, these are now uncommon.

ECT remains a contentious issue, and current controversies will be considered in more detail in Chapter 18. Nevertheless, many nurses will be impressed by the improvement they see in patients who have undergone the treatment. Nurses have a clearly defined role to play in ensuring their patients' well-being, prior to, during and after the administration of ECT.

Pre-ECT care

Most people nowadays are aware of the existence of ECT and consequently, on entering a psychiatric hospital, will realise they may possibly be offered this form of treatment.

Depending on their preconceived ideas, they may dread it, doggedly refuse to consider it, or actively seek it out. Irrespective of prejudice, however, anyone about to undergo ECT will be anxious. This is an understandable and perfectly normal response when faced with an unknown experience involving a general anaesthetic.

Although there are few contraindications to ECT, the patient will have been given a strict physical examination, prior to having it prescribed. Recent heart trouble, brittle bones, or a propensity to dementia would most likely rule out ECT. In situations where patients with these conditions were, because of the real risk of suicide, in a life-threatening situation, the consultant psychiatrist would have to carefully weigh up all the pros and cons before reaching a decision. A patient unable to withstand the rigours of general anaesthesia, would be unlikely to be treated, as straight ECT is almost never considered.

An informal patient must give his consent, which should be informed consent. The doctor must give a careful explanation of the treatment, and sign the appropriate section of the form, stating he has done so.

A patient undergoing treatment under a section of the Mental Health Act may on occasion, be treated against his will. Certain safeguards, including a second doctor's opinion and the need to seek the views of others, such as the nurse, must be adhered to, before proceeding with treatment in these circumstances. Needless to say, the active co-operation of the patient makes for a more pleasant experience all round, and may possibly even make a successful outcome more likely.

The nurse should make herself familiar with the way the doctor carries out his explanation. She will often be approached by an anxious patient who may have forgotten what he has been told, or who is seeking confirmation on a certain point. Any apparent discrepancy between the opinion or advice of different members of staff may have the unfortunate effect of escalating the patient's anxiety level. Staff with a positive opinion of ECT are more likely to impart a spirit of optimism which will be transmitted to their patients.

On the evening prior to ECT, a sedative may be prescribed to ensure a good night's sleep. Since treatment normally takes place in the forenoon, the patient will be advised that he must fast over breakfast, in preparation for the anaesthetic.

The morning of the treatment will be an anxious time for the patient. In a well-staffed ward, one nurse may be allocated his care, and should provide empathic support and diversion. Advantage should be taken of the fortuitous presence of another patient in the ward who has experienced ECT and who no longer fears it. He may be able to impart a degree of reassurance that the nurse cannot provide.

Half an hour before treatment, *a premedication*, usually atropine, will be given if prescribed. This relaxes smooth muscle and dries up secretions, but to be effective, it must be given at exactly the right time. Many anaesthetists now prefer to administer the atropine intravenously, immediately prior to the treatment and the nurse is thus relieved of the responsibility.

A well-orchestrated approach is essential to ensure treatment starts at the stated time. Prolonged waiting after this will be doubly upsetting.

Anyone who has ever waited in a dentist's queue will appreciate the need for promptness, and also the fact that incidental noises from other patients' treatment should take place out of earshot. It is important that there should be two doors in the treatment room so that any post-ECT confusion in an earlier patient is not witnessed by those waiting.

Patients having ECT do not require to undress, but neckties should be removed, restrictive belts and clothing loosened and the feet exposed.

The patient should visit the toilet in order to empty his bladder and bowels, thus avoiding the embarrassing and unnecessary possibility of incontinence occurring during treatment.

Prosthesis should be removed, and any valuables or personal jewellery should be given to the nurse for safekeeping.

A minority of psychiatric patients may be unsure of their identity or highly suspicious of those around them. The loss of their valued, personal cues may increase these tendencies, so the understanding nurse will wait until the last possible minute before removing them, returning them as soon as the patient is able to resume responsibility once again.

The management of ECT

The patient will be taken to the treatment room, or alternatively, the means of administering the treatment will be wheeled to his bedside. Either way, care should be taken not to expose the patient to the sight of strange equipment, at a time when he will be at his most vulnerable.

The patient will be assisted on to a padded table, or encouraged to lie down in bed, and a light, short-acting, general anaesthetic is administered by intravenous injection. This will probably either be methohexitone or thiopentone. A muscle relaxant, such as suxamethonium, will be given immediately afterwards.

The anaesthetic must always precede the muscle relaxant, because the sensation of being totally relaxed (including the muscles of respiration) is extremely frightening for someone who is conscious.

The administration of these drugs by the anaesthetist is a considerable refinement of the treatment in its original form and makes for an experience altogether less spectacular or terrifying.

The patient is then ventilated with oxygen, and a mouth gag is placed between the teeth. A pre-set dose of electricity, which is sufficient to cause a convulsion, is then administered via the two electrodes which are held by the psychiatrist, in position on the patient's head.

At this point, a violent clenching of the jaw will be observed, although other muscles will stiffen only slightly. This is due to the fact that the electricity flows directly through the muscles of the jaw, and muscle relaxants are ineffective against such direct stimulation.

Where adequate muscle relaxant is used, the firm, but gentle, holding of the lower jaw against the mouth gag is the only restraint that may be necessary.

No dramatic thrashing of limbs or foaming at the mouth takes place, the only evidence of a convulsion, frequently being the characteristic contracted appearance of the toes, which are exposed purely for this reason.

As soon as the doctor is satisfied that a fit has taken place, the mouth gag is removed and an airway reinserted. Oxygen or air via an ambu bag is then given by the anaesthetist, until the patient recommences spontaneous breathing.

Patients are then placed in the semi-prone position, and handed over to the care of a trained nurse. **Close observation**, as for all post-anaesthetic patients is required, until consciousness is recovered. This usually occurs in less than 15 minutes.

In the treatment room the nurse's duties are to re-assure the patient prior to anaesthesia, to ensure the equipment is readily available and in working order, and possibly to apply gentle restraint to the lower jaw.

Post-ECT care

Routine post-ECT care falls within the sphere of nursing competence, although they should immediately summon the anaesthetist should they suspect even the hint of a complication.

While the patient is still unconscious, the maintenance of a clear **airway** is a priority. A careful check should be made for vomiting or cyanosis.

Consciousness will be recovered quickly but the patient may be suffering from transient confusion and will certainly have no memory of the event. The presence of a familiar face at this time can be reassuring, and typically, the patient will wish to roll over and doze to an uneventful recovery.

While serving the tea and toast in lieu of the missed breakfast, the nurse should take the opportunity of tact-fully addressing everyone by name, thus helping the process of orientation.

If a headache results after consciousness is regained, it will normally be treated with paracetamol or as-pirin, unless they are contraindicated. **Unexpected sequelae**, such as marked confusion, severe headache, or undue drowsiness, should be reported, as they may in-fluence any decision as to when treatment should be discontinued.

If given to an outpatient, careful observation is required to ensure that he is fit to leave the safety of the hospital. In such cases, he should always be **accompanied** by a friend or relative.

At one time it was considered normal to give a complete 'course' of six treatments in almost every case. Although this number still represents an average, the more sensible approach of reviewing progress after each treatment, and proceeding accordingly, is now widespread. This guards against the possibility of a sudden mood swing, as overtreatment can occasionally precipitate a manic reaction.

The nurse should be aware that someone recovering from a severe depression represents a **serious suicidal risk**. Often he will experience an upsurge of energy and drive, before his depressive thoughts disappear. While previously he may have lacked the direction to put suicidal thoughts into action, this now becomes a distinct possibility. The decision, therefore, to relax observation on a recovering patient, who was thought to have suicidal tendencies, is never taken lightly.

ECT given as described along with a muscle relaxant, is termed 'modified' ECT and side-effects are rare. However, some memory impairment seems inevitable, causing alarm in many prospective patients.

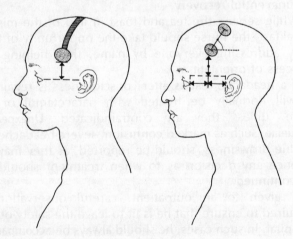

Fig. 6.1 Bilateral ECT (left) and unilateral ECT (right).

Unilateral ECT (Fig. 6.1), where both electrodes are applied to the same side of the head and the current passes through the non-dominant hemisphere of the brain, reduces substantially the degree of memory impairment and may prove to be just as effective as the original *bilateral* method, involving both temples (Fig. 6.1).

Mrs W. (54 years old), had spent a lifetime free of major psychiatric symptoms. According to her husband and two daughters, her lifestyle had been normal, if a trifle humdrum. She, herself, made little comment.

During the past year, Mrs W. had changed dramatically. Despite regular visits to her GP she had sunk into a deep depression which culminated in her admission to hospital following an extremely serious drug overdose. She expressed the belief that she was too sinful to live, and that she had 'betrayed' her religion.

This tendency for some people to develop severe depressive symptoms for the first time during the years of middle age is well recognised. In the past it was colourfully described as '*involutional melancholia*', a term which now seems to have all but disappeared.

With drug therapy already having proved ineffective and Mrs W.'s life being in grave danger, ECT would have been considered immediately. During an interview with the psychiatrist, Mr and Mrs W. were given a description of ECT and asked to consent to treatment. They may have been relieved to hear that the prognosis in such illnesses is usually favourable.

Mrs W., encouraged by her husband, signed the form.

Staff are accustomed to nursing people like Mrs W. and her treatment was dramatic, only in its outcome. Seven ECT's were given over the course of a month, resulting in an almost complete recovery.

With her husband, Mrs W. left the hospital, displaying a degree of purposefulness and optimism, that she had previously imagined were gone forever. She had been in hospital for just 2 months.

Of course, other factors may have influenced Mrs W.'s recovery. The hospital environment, the ward meetings, the cyclical nature of affective disorders, or the placebo effect of hospitalisation and being taken seriously, may all have played a part. Nervertheless, ECT's apparent contribution should not be minimised.

The least it may have done is pulled Mrs W. back from the edge of her personal precipice, allowing her to avail herself of the other facilities on offer. This is a *life-saving property*, and one which it consistently achieves.

Staff are familiar with many such success stories, which despite certain well-publicised misgivings, seems to ensure a continued place in psychiatry for ECT.

CHEMOTHERAPY

The other main form of physical treatment is chemotherapy — the use of drugs.

As a result of new drugs which are constantly being marketed, changing fashions and doctors who insist on prescribing their personal favourites, it is impossible to catalogue every drug the nurse may be asked to administer.

What follows, therefore, is an introduction to *psychotrophic drugs*, (drugs that alter feeling, perception and behaviour, without significantly altering consciousness), and the examples mentioned are precisely that.

Major tranquillisers

The introduction of major tranquillising drugs in the early 1950s is arguably the most significant event this century as far as psychiatric nursing is concerned.

These drugs calm the patient down, without making him fall asleep. They are useful in controlling overactive behaviour, and seem to have a directly modifying effect on the hallucinations and delusions of some psychotic individuals.

The first major tranquilliser was chlorpromazine (Largactil) and it remains popular today. It is a member of the *phenothiazene* group of drugs, which also include the widely prescribed thioridazine and trifluperazine. The latter is said to have a particularly effective antihallucinogenic property, and is commonly used in cases of acute and chronic schizophrenia.

Haloperidol is not a phenothiazene, but shares similar features, and is another useful major tranquilliser.

Important and influential as these drugs are, they have several side-effects. These include Parkinsonian features of facial rigidity and stiffness of the limbs, which respond to anti-Parkinsonian drugs such as orphenadrine.

Typically, a 'pill-rolling' motion of the thumb on the palm of the hand can be observed, while more seriously, a *dyskenesia*, which seems to be irreversible, occasionally develops. This involves continual, distressing, oro-facial contortions and grimacing, which are not relieved by treatment. The use of the tranquilliser responsible should be discontinued.

Other important side-effects are jaundice and, very uncommonly, agranulocytosis. (Although extremely rare, this should be borne in mind, if the patient complains of a sore throat.)

It has become common to use depot, that is *long-acting* tranquillisers such as flupenthixol decanoate, or fluphenazine decanoate (Modecate) in the treatment of schizophrenia.

Although these preparations have the obvious advantage that they need only be taken once every 2, 3 or 4 weeks, they have no influence on the incidence of side-effects.

Some patients, especially those taking chlorpromazine, will be very sensitive to the sun. This is important when planning nursing care, since they should never be allowed into the sunshine, unless suitably protected by a cream or a sun hat.

Winter, too, may bring its problems, and in the elderly, the possibility of hypothermia should be considered, since the temperature-regulating ability of the body tends to become less efficient.

Chlorpromazine can cause contact dermatitis and nurses giving it by injection, or whose skin may be especially sensitive, should wear gloves for their protection.

> John had been a great problem to hospital staff during his younger days. Fit and strong, he had worked in the hospital farm, when not locked up because of his violent and unpredictable behaviour. He could never leave the hospital grounds, unless heavily escorted, which was of course, usually impossible.
>
> John has been on major tranquillisers for many years now. Today, he receives an injection every 3 weeks, and although he must remain an inpatient, he has free access to the nearby town. He takes an anti-Parkinsonian drug three times a day, for his moderate side-effects.
>
> John's condition is not 'cured', nor will it ever be, but major tranquillisers have changed his lifestyle.
>
> Like so many others, he can now enjoy the facilities available to him and he has regained his self-respect, which was missing during his long violent battles with staff.

Minor tranquillisers

These drugs, of which diazepam (Valium) and chlordiazepoxide are commonly used examples, are widely prescribed for the treatment of anxiety states.

Although previously considered to be safe, they potentiate the effects of alcohol, and may interfere with the ability to drive, or operate machinery. More recently concern has been expressed about the prolonged use of minor tranquillisers, since it has been established that dependency can readily occur. Dizziness and ataxia is often seen in elderly users and may be upsetting enough to make them reach for yet another tablet to relieve their anxiety.

A pleasing feature of these drugs is their safety, when taken as an overdose, since fatalities are unheard of.

Antidepressant drugs

Of all the psychotrophic drugs, we understand perhaps most clearly, how these appear to work. Mood is related to the concentration of amines, such as noradrenaline and 5-hydroxytryptamine in the brain, a reduction of which leads to a depressed mood.

Antidepressant drugs are classified into three main groups:

(i) Tricyclics
(ii) Tetracyclics
(iii) Monoamine oxidase inhibitors (MAOIs).

Tricyclics

These increase the level of amines and are the most popular antidepressants in current use. Examples include imipramine and amitriptyline, while a sustained release version of amitriptyline (Lentizol) is useful, in that it need be taken only once daily in the evening, when it may also help promote sleep.

Side-effects include, dryness of the mouth, blurring of vision, constipation, states of excitement and hypotension.

Although widely prescribed, an important property of these drugs is the fact that they take 2–3 weeks to reach their maximum efficiency. This may involve an unacceptable suicide risk.

Tetracyclics

A relatively new development, the tetracyclics display a similar action to the tricyclics. Mianserin (Bolvidon) is a tetracyclic drug that is commonly prescribed.

Monoamine oxidase inhibitors (MAOIs)

Monoamine oxidase is an enzyme responsible for the

breakdown of amines in nerve endings in the brain. By blocking this enzyme, MAOIs cause an accumulation of amines and when successful, a corresponding rise in spirits.

These drugs are not always effective but seem to be occasionally successful in very resistive depressions. Normally they are tried, only after ECT and tricyclics have failed to work.

This is partly due to the fact that if taken in conjunction with tyramine-containing foods such as cheese, yoghurt, alcohol, broad beans, meat extracts (Bovril), yeast extracts (Marmite), or the tricyclic type antidepressant, a severe hypertensive reaction can result. While the need to stick to such a diet may prove mildly irritating while a patient is in hospital, it may become almost impossible after discharge.

Phenelzine is an example of a MAOI.

Lithium

Used prophylactically, lithium produces a stabilising effect on the mood and is important in the long-term management of manic depressive psychosis and recurrent endogenous depression.

Since toxicity occurs at a plasma concentration level only a little higher than the therapeutic dose, a careful check, involving regular medical follow-up, must be kept on plasma concentration levels. Polyuria, polydipsia and weight gain may occur even when the correct doseage is taken, but raised plasma levels can produce hypothyroidism, drowsiness, coarse tremors, vomiting, diarrhoea, dysarthria or even coma and death. Any indication of those more serious side-effects would result in the drug being immediately withdrawn.

Patients with a history of recurring manic depression may require a life-long maintenance dose of lithium.

Chemotherapy and the nurse

Complicated as the chemical action of drugs may be, this is only part of the story. Many people will react to any tablet they may be given, whether or not it contains an active ingredient. This so-called 'placebo effect' may explain many dramatic improvements. The attitude of the nurse dispensing the tablet is also important. A nurse who strongly believes in the drug will transmit some of her optimism to the patient, who may then react favourably.

A nurse in a psychiatric ward shares with her general colleagues, all the responsibilities of ensuring that the correct patient receives the correct dose of the correct drug, at the correct time but sometimes this may prove difficult.

Psychiatric patients do not as a rule wear identity bracelets, which could be seen as stigma-provoking, and are rarely confined to bed. Yet some may be unable, or unwilling to identify themselves.

Ocassionally, patients will refuse medication on the grounds that they do not think that they are ill, while others may fear that they are being poisoned. It is important, however, to realise that all refusals to take medicine cannot be explained away as a psychiatric symptom. Most drugs have side-effects and some patients, rather than report any unexpected sensations, may decide to stop taking them. Others too, will dislike the taste, or have difficulty in swallowing tablets, but once this is realised it can usually be rectified by having it prescribed in a different form.

A minority of patients will pretend to take the drug, but will in fact try to save it for use in a future suicide bid. Here, more than anywhere, the rule that patients must be *seen* to swallow their tablet is paramount. The simple tactic of getting the patient to speak once the drug is in his mouth will usually reveal whether or not it has been swallowed.

Observing the effects of drug treatment

The nurse must carefully observe the patients to whom she has given medication. Improvements will be gratifying but side-effects are equally likely. It is important that the nurse's preconceived ideas do not affect her judgement, and that she reports exactly what she sees.

Drug therapy has revolutionised many aspects of psychiatric nursing, but should not be seen as a be-all and end-all. If the strait-jackets of yesteryear are replaced merely by the chemical strait-jacket of today's powerful drugs, we have advanced little. Rather, the strength of chemotherapy should be seen as its ability to dampen the patient's more florid symptoms. This means that they become available for the battery of psychological and environmental therapies, which along with drugs, may eventually combine to favourably influence the outcome of treatment.

PSYCHOSURGERY — LEUCOTOMY

At one time, surgery was a commonly used method of modifying the symptoms of psychiatric illness but it was largely superseded by ECT and later, the tranquillisers.

Although techniques have now been greatly refined, there remains many moral as well as clinical objections to its use. At present psychosurgery seems to be confined to a tiny handful of patients, crippled by anxiety and tension, with perhaps obsessive compulsive features which have failed completely to respond to other forms of treatment. It is possible that as the procedure becomes increasingly sophisticated and our knowledge of the brain expands, some people may clamour for the reinstatement of leucotomy as a widely available alternative.

CHANGING FASHIONS IN PHYSICAL TREATMENT

The history of physical methods of treatment in psychiatry is long and while we can perhaps disregard the instruments and restraints of bygone centuries, it is noteworthy that treatments popular, even a short while ago, are now no longer used. *Deep insulin comas* are a thing of the past. Even *modified insulin therapy*, an essential feature in most recent texts on physical methods of psychiatric treatment, can now almost be ignored. Along with continuous or *prolonged narcosis* ('the sleep cure') it has slipped from relevance over the past decade or so.

SUGGESTED READING

Connechen J, Robson H, Shanley E 1983 Pharmacology for nurses. Nurses' Aids Series. Bailliére Tindall, London

Chapter 18 may be read in conjunction with this chapter.

7

Psychologically-orientated treatment

One reason for the mystique surrounding psychiatry and psychiatrists may be the knowledge that they sometimes treat their patients by 'just talking'. If attempts at cure by operation or the passing of electricity through the brain are mysterious, achieving the same end merely through the spoken word seems almost magical. Success in some people's eyes would elevate the psychiatrist to a par with Jesus Christ or an African Witch Doctor.

There is nothing magical about psychotherapy as the talking cure is officially known. Any patient who anticipates lying back and enjoying an instant cure without any effort or hardship on his part is doomed to instant disappointment. A quest for such a painless solution, however, may be behind some people's insistence on being treated with hypnosis or the 'truth drug', and their surprise that such methods are not used more frequently.

Hypnosis

Hypnosis has a strictly limited role in modern psychiatry but is important historically. It was used in the early part of the 18th century by a flamboyant Austrian physician, *T. A. Mesmer* (from whom we get the word mesmerise) who developed an elaborate theory called animal magnetism. Through this theory he sought to explain how one person could influence the thoughts or deeds of another. He suggested this was achieved by the passing of some kind of 'invisible fluid' between the two participants, and it is not surprising therefore that his theory fell into disrepute.

However, by the latter part of the 19th century, the renowned neurologist, Charcot, was using hypnosis extensively. Eventually he was joined by a student, Sigmund Freud, who was to change completely the understanding of personality development and the treatment of some forms of psychological distress. His influence remains potent, even today.

Intially Freud relied on hypnosis to prompt his patients to recall long forgotten childhood incidents, which he considered were crucial in the development of their current distress. Shortly we shall see how Freud discarded hypnosis in favour of other techniques, although the aims of his treatment remained similar.

Today the use of hypnosis in psychiatry is strictly limited, although the nurse may be involved in relaxation techniques which are based on a form of modified hypnosis.

Some patients who, like Freud's earlier examples, appear to suffer from a hysterical condition manifested by a physical symptom for instance a paralysed limb, could have their actual symptom removed by a skilled hypnotist. This is fraught with dangers, however, as the conflicts originally responsible for the symptoms remain. Denied his (unconsciously selected) prop, the patient may relapse, develop alternative symptoms or even in extreme cases, commit suicide.

Martin had represented his country at soccer at both schoolboy and youth level. On signing professional forms, he was deemed to have a glittering career ahead of him. Sadly he seemed to be plagued by injuries, particularly to his right knee. It refused to respond to a variety of treatments including surgery, and eventually acupuncture.

After several private sessions with a hypnotist, Martin's knee was completely 'cured', but inexplicably he began to drink heavily shortly afterwards. Now, several years later as his short career nears its end, it is obvious that Martin will not make it 'big'. He plays for a third rate outfit but enjoys a local reputation as the one who would have reached the very top but for his unfortunate addiction to alcohol.

More recently he has been attending a psychiatrist and for the first time, believes he can explain his checkered existence. Martin faces the fact that, from an early age, he had been unconsciously aware that he did not quite have the talent to maintain his early promise. His injury protected him from acknowledging the fact that he could only ever be an average professional, and even brought him a lot of sympathy.

Martin's 'cure' in no way examined his inner conflicts and may even have fostered vague ideas that he was somehow a fraud. His alcoholism (possibly a more serious condition) merely took over, and nothing permanent was achieved.

Nowadays hypnosis's main contribution to medicine is not in the psychiatric field but in *obstetrics*, *dentistry* and *painful terminal illness*. Here patients can be taught to relax in relative comfort, while analgesia if required can be given in greatly reduced doses.

Abreaction

When used properly this term describes the release to the conscious of material that has previously been repressed. When the psychiatrist considers that it could be helpful, he may facilitate this response by the intravenous injection of a drug such as Pentothal. Thus in popular usage, the term abreaction has come to be applied to both the release of repressed material and less accurately, to the specialised method of bringing it about.

This is the 'truth drug' beloved by American film writers. It may enable the patient to relive with vivid clarity a particularly disturbing or stressful experience in his early childhood which had hitherto been completely repressed. This recall is helped by the relaxing properties of the drug which allows the patient to feel less inhibited about stating what is on his mind. Some psychotherapists find it useful when treatment has reached an impasse and the patient cannot produce any more material unaided. Readers who may have had too much to drink at a party may recall a similar situation, where they spoke freely about a subject which they would normally find inhibiting. In treatment as at parties, there is no guarantee that the material thus produced is the truth. In fact it seems likely that unfettered by normal morality, some people may well let their imaginations run riot. Like hypnosis this is a treatment of limited value but it may be successful with the occasional patient who is proving difficult to treat.

Hypnosis and drug-assisted abreaction have a special appeal to somewhat immature individuals who want treatment to be something that is done *to* them. They may say, or more often imply, 'Here I am doctor (or nurse), you make me better.'

The road to recovery is never that easy. Psychotherapy involves the patient in long and emotionally powerful sessions in which the bulk of the work is done by him. We shall now explore some of the more common forms of psychotherapy.

PSYCHOTHERAPY

Psychoanalysis

The term psychoanalysis is used in two distinct contexts. Firstly, it describes the theory of personality development first described by Freud which forms the basis of much of Chapter 9. Also, it describes a method of psychological treatment, again first practised by Freud.

Freud stated that mental functioning could be divided into three levels: the *conscious*, the *preconscious* and the *unconscious*. All that we are aware of at a given time comprises the conscious, while the much larger amount of facts or images that we can produce at will makes up the preconscious. We do not go around constantly aware of the F. A. Cup Winners of 1953 or of the theorem of Pythagoras, but if asked, many of us could recall these and an incalculable amount of other facts almost instantaneously.

The unconscious mind is made up of memories, desires and conflicts of which we are not aware, and of which we cannot become aware even by a deliberate effort of will.

Freud found that under hypnosis many of his patients could recall previously forgotten material, often of a frightening or sexual nature and furthermore, those whose newly-acquired recall was most acute, seemed to make the best improvement. Eventually he stopped using hypnosis (partly it is said because he wasn't very good at it) and concentrated instead on the techniques of *dream interpretation* and *free association*. In free association patients were encouraged to speak of any subject that came to mind, however bizzare or apparently irrelevant, while the doctor or psychoanalyst as he was called said very little. Freud considered that the closer topics came to areas that were emotionally charged, the more difficulty the patient experienced in talking freely. As the months passed it became possible for the analyst to suggest various events or people from the patient's past that had had an important influence on their mental development.

Also of crucial importance to Freud's theory was the concept of *transference* (Ch. I). This is the tendency to attribute feelings and attitudes experienced towards some significant person in the past to someone in a current interpersonal relationship. Thus the therapist may become the recipient of love or hate which was previously felt for a parent or sibling many years before. Often there will be a mixture of both these feelings, a state known as *ambivalence*. By working through and coming to understand their current relation with their analysts, patients (clients) may gain valuable insight into their personalities, and characteristic methods of relating to people.

Psychoanalysis does not as a rule discover one all important, horrific experience which can explain all that happens thereafter, nor does the therapist spend much time trying to convert the client to his viewpoint. Nevertheless, psychoanalysis is the most ambitious form of psychological treatment currently available and aims to reconstruct completely the individual's personality.

Pscyhoanalysis is extremely expensive, partly because it involves hourly sessions four or five times a week for up to 5 years, and partly because, before he can practise each analyst must himself be analysed. It is not available through the National Health Service. People receiving psychoanalysis are not usually inpatients, but require to be highly motivated and likely to persevere with treatment even during the inevitable periods of disillusionment.

The nurse, therefore, is unlikely to come across a patient who is receiving psychoanalysis but the principles of the treatment are still important. The concepts of the unconscious, of uninterrupted free speech and of transference have been borrowed from psychoanalysis and play an important part in most psychotherapies practised today.

Psychotherapy is the treatment of choice for individuals who display neurotic symptoms, (Ch. II) or whose main problems lie in an inability to relate adequately to others.

Individual psychotherapy

Individual psychotherapy involves many interviews with a therapist (usually a psychiatrist) over a lengthy period of time. Most people who undergo psychotherapy do so as outpatients, although they may commence therapy as an in patient, or may require a short period of hospitalisation during a particularly traumatic stage of treatment.

In analytical psychotherapy, the patient explores with the therapist his past and current relationships. Free association and interpretation of dreams may be used depending on the orientation of the therapist, and the transference situation will be explored.

The aim of the therapy is to provide insight and highlight areas of unhealthy mental functioning in the patient. The cornerstone of this approach is the theory that once a symptom has been explained it will become unnecessary and will be discarded leaving the individual more capable of relating maturely to his surroundings. Its opponents would claim that this does not necessarily happen.

It is generally assumed that for analytical psychotherapy to be most successful, the patient (client) should be young(ish), above average intelligence, articulate and determined to continue in treatment.

Supportive psychotherapy

Sometimes, the patient may be none of these things, or for some entirely different reason may be considered unsuitable for analytical therapy.

Marilyn (40 years old) was below average intelligence and her three children (born in close succession) were rapidly growing up. She was short, plump and rather unattractive and seemed to be the object of thinly veiled contempt from her husband and family. She was not an interesting or rewarding person to have around.

Amazingly, despite inadequate domestic or budgeting skills, Marilyn, over the years, had just managed to get by.

However, an accumulation of financial problems, an extra-marital affair of the husband and her children's increasing independence were threatening to overwhelm her. After an initial assessment, Marilyn's therapy was allocated to a specially experienced nurse. The plan was not ambitious but merely aimed at helping her re-establish her previous coping mechanisms.

In the event it proved highly successful. For probably the first time Marilyn was taken seriously. Her therapist's warmth and encouragement provided her with a new experience. For once she could talk to someone who seemed prepared to listen. Little has changed for Marilyn but once again she is getting by. Realistically this is the best that can be expected and the therapist must now concentrate on weaning her from treatment before she becomes over dependent.

Damage can be done by attempting to explore the unconscious of people like Marilyn. Often their grip on normality may be so tenuous that too much probing may render them acutely disturbed. The aim is to shore up rather than break down their usual defence mechanisms, allowing them to function very much as their pre-crisis self. The therapist, who implies that (perhaps for the first time) what they say really matters, may greatly boost their morale and that may prove to be all the treatment that is required.

Group psychotherapy

Psychotherapy is time-consuming and trained therapists are relatively few in number. This means that only a limited amount of individuals, capable of benefiting from psychotherapy, can hope to receive treatment at any one time. Logically, the principles of psychotherapy were introduced to the group setting, and group psychotherapy was developed. It soon became apparent that group psychotherapy was more than just a watered down version of individual psychotherapy, proving for some people, to be the treatment of choice.

A group can consist of any number of individuals, but probably between five and twelve is ideal. Because of the fact that several people make up a group a wide variety of behaviour or symptoms will be on display at any one time. This may have the effect of persuading the patient that his problems are not unique and may give him encouragement to battle on. Some members may be unwilling to accept the norms of the therapist whom they consider to be different or out of touch, but may pay attention to their peers.

By its ability to reward its members by warmth and encouragement or conversely, to punish them by rejection, the group can exert a tremendous pressure on any individual member to conform to its collective standards. This may account for its apparent success in dealing with some patients who are described as having a personality disorder.

Most groups will have a formal leader, who may be any one of the staff team, and perhaps a co-leader. However, as the group dynamics enfold, the nurse may become aware of someone else, probably a patient, vying for the informal leadership of the group. If the formal leadership of the group is weak, they may succeed.

Scapegoating, when the group focuses on one member in a negative way and blames him for everything that has gone wrong, is a feature of some groups. The likelihood of this happening is enhanced if one group member stands out in any obvious way. It is not a good idea for instance to have one female, one homosexual, one black person, or one member of the working class in a group.

Collusion, when a number of patients appear to make an unspoken pact to thwart the aims of the group is common, and when in evidence, should be brought out in to the open. Undercurrents of anger, fear or distrust can sometimes be detected in the group as a whole and may be of an intensity equal to anything that individual psychotherapy can throw up.

A group may be *open* — patients joining or leaving it as their symptoms vary — or *closed* — where everyone joins it together and continues without additions until its planned disbandment.

They may, depending on the needs of their members and orientation of the therapist, be merely supportive, (the so-called tea and sympathy group), intensely analytical, or anything in between.

Family therapy, marital therapy, psychodrama

There are many psychological methods of treatment of which the above are purely examples. Many are loosely based on psychotherapeutic principles, and all aim to encourage more mature living patterns in those seeking help.

One psychological treatment, however, seems to contradict directly many of the principles cited above.

BEHAVIOUR THERAPY

Behaviour therapy describes a number of treatments which are based on the so-called learning theory. *Behaviourists*, as people who use behaviour therapy are known, believe that psychiatric symptoms arise as a result of faulty learning. Consequently, they believe patients can re-learn more acceptable habits, or unlearn the ones that are giving rise to concern.

In stark contrast to psychoanalytical reasoning, behaviourists make no attempt to unravel complicated details from their patient's past. This they would see as an unnecessarily irrelevant piece of self-indulgent nonsense. Instead, their only interest is the patient's observable behaviour, which they claim can be moulded satisfactorily using learning techniques.

Mothers will be aware of the effect that a reward can have in encouraging desired behaviour in her children. This is the philosophy behind the frequently heard plea of 'eat up your vegetables, then you can have your sweet'. Behaviourists would call the sweet a *'reinforcer'* and given immediately following the observed behaviour of eating vegetables, it will mean that vegetables are more likely to be eaten in the future. Of course not all reinforcers need be tangible, and approval in the form of a smile or a hug from mother will frequently have the desired effect on a small child.

Should undesirable behaviour require to be eradicated, the mother may smack her child, i.e. punish it, or withdraw a reinforcer. For instance, we may be told of an attention seeking infant, 'Ignore him and he will soon stop.' This is sound advice.

Token economy

Sometimes whole wards are run on this principle and are known as token economy wards. Patients who are usually institutionalised will have a programme of goals established and immediately one of them is achieved they will be given a token. This can later be exchanged for goods or privileges which they desire. These tokens are reinforcers and will increase the likelihood of the desired behaviour being repeated, in much the same way as gift coupons encourage smokers to buy a particular brand of cigarettes. When the desired behaviour is not achieved tokens must be withheld.

Remarkable improvements have been reported in some 'chronic' wards following the introduction of token economy schemes with mutism, incontinence and deplorable personal hygiene all proving amenable to treatment. All hospital staff should be aware that a token economy programme is in operation but the role of the nurse in particular is absolutely vital. She must be completely familiar with the programme and consistent in what she reinforces. A nurse, who because of a mistaken sense of kindness gives a token when it has not been earned, or one who cannot be bothered to reward a desired piece of behaviour, can do untold damage to the treatment plan.

A problem for some nurses is that they may unwittingly reinforce undesireable behaviour and so exacerbate the very symptoms they would like to see eradicated.

Robin (54 years old) has been a patient for most of the last 30 years. By far the bulk of this time has been spent in a soulless 50-bedded ward with only basic facilities.

The outstanding feature of Robin's condition was a bizarre delusional system incorporating such diversities as H. Bombs, mosquitoes, penguins and aborigines! Furthermore, it was his custom to talk incessantly about them to all who cared to listen.

Over the years, as new members of staff or various interested parties were introduced to the ward, they were invariably approached by Robin, giving vent to his particular delusion of the day. Staff overlooked or tacitly encouraged these interventions, presumably on the rather dubious grounds that they were frankly amusing, and that they provided an ideal teaching situation, being a classical, though particularly florid example of paranoid schizophrenia.

A new charge nurse on his arrival in the ward spotted that Robin's bizarre behaviour made him the centre of attraction — a positive reinforcer. Alternatively, if he acted 'normally' he would fade into the background, along with his 40 fellow patients and could literally be unnoticed. The charge nurse instructed that from then on bizzare talk had to be politely but firmly ignored, while his occasional rational conversation had to be responded to with warmth and interest.

Robin's habits were too ingrained to be completely eradicated, but it was interesting that once the desired rather than the undesired behaviour was rewarded, the incidence of delusional utterances diminished appreciably.

Aversion therapy

One type of therapy which has received more than its fair share of publicity is aversion therapy. This was first used in the 1930s and although self mutilation, gambling, deviant sexual behaviour and alcoholism might all respond, most work was done with alcoholics.

This was done by injecting the individual with a drug (usually apomorphine) and then presenting him with his favourite tipple; as this happened, the drug caused him to vomit. Thus by pairing vomiting with the presentation of alcohol, the hope was that the sight and smell of alcohol would eventually be sufficient to produce nausea, and the urge to drink would be diminished.

When behaviour which may bring the patient into conflict with the police is treated, this will usually involve the patient in merely imagining his particular deviation in great detail (to carry it out may be illegal or degrading), and again an unpleasant stimulus, this time usually an electric shock will be administered.

Since this treatment is uncomfortable and possibly dangerous, patients agreeing to undergo it must be physically fit and highly motivated. Even so, results are patchy and it seems that some people respond for a limited period only. To remain symptom-free they have to present themselves for 'topping up' treatment at regular intervals.

Although used fairly infrequently, aversion therapy may arouse strong emotions in a nurse who witnesses it. Nurses give many reasons for wanting to enter the profession, but the wish to inflict calculated unpleasantness on their patients is not usually one of them. Some will consider aversion therapy to be in direct conflict with their caring principles.

Systematic desensitisation

Sometimes known as *reciprocal inhibition*, this treatment

is widely used. It enjoys a better reputation among the detractors of behaviour therapy than does other methods. Used as a treatment for anxiety the aim of the therapist is to induce a feeling of placidity and relaxation in the patient. As such feelings are incompatible with the anxious state, the patient when fully relaxed is gradually introduced to the frightening stimulus.

It is particularly effective in the treatment of the so-called monosymptomatic phobia, when someone with a reasonably integrated personality displays an irrational fear of one specific situation.

Mary (23 years old) had always been outgoing and popular, but promotion at work had highlighted a hitherto unsuspected problem. Her new job demanded that she travelled frequently to Europe and Mary, it transpired, was terrified of flying.

Eventually, it was decided that Mary should be treated by desensitisation under the auspices of a clinical psychologist. First, Mary was taught to relax completely, using a cassette recording borrowed from her therapist, the psychologist. Then she had to make out a list of all her feared situations relating to flying. She had to arrange them in order starting with the least frightening and going on to the most terrifying. This list is called a *hierarchy*.

Mary then had to bring about a state of relaxation before facing up to the first step in the hierarchy — handling a toy aeroplane belonging to her nephew. After each session she was asked to rate her anxiety level and she could proceed to the next stage only when this was minimal. Gradually as each step in the hierarchy was achieved she came closer to her final ambition — to go unaccompanied to the airport and board a plane. Mary no longer attends for therapy but recently her therapist received a postcard from Malta, where she had flown on holiday!

This gradual introduction of the relaxed patient to the feared stimulus enjoys some success, and Mary's case seemed particularly suited to it. Her phobia was very specific; she was also young, intelligent and apparently otherwise well-adjusted, but above all, she genuinely wanted to change.

Flooding

Not all phobias are treated by desensitisation. In fact a technique which seems almost its exact opposite is sometimes employed. This is called flooding or *implosion* and involves confronting the patient with his most feared situation immediately, on the assumption, no doubt that if he survives that, he will survive anything!

Thus a woman afraid of crowds would be taken to the supermarket on a Saturday morning and left to find her own way home. Believers in this method of treatment claim that it is much quicker than desensitisation, and that relapses are less likely. Nevertheless before this method is employed it is necessary for the patient to be physically fit and highly motivated.

Behaviour therapy — a criticism

Behaviour therapy has attracted a lot of support and a good deal of criticism. Unfortunately psychiatry has tended to split into two camps, the psychoanalytical and the behaviourist, and sadly each claim to see little merit in the other's ideas. Behaviour therapy is good in that results may come about fairly quickly and since it is actual behaviour that is modified, changes can be readily seen and measured.

The inescapable criticism of behaviour therapy which is loudly cited by its detractors is the fact that the reasons for any piece of behaviour are quite deliberately ignored. As with Martin and his hypnosis, the underlying conflict remains unaltered and a relapse or the occurrence of a completely new set of symptoms must be a possibility.

THE ROLE OF THE NURSE IN PSYCHOLOGICAL TREATMENTS

Since many types of psychotherapy are largely a private

concern between the patient and his therapist, nurses may tend to feel rather left out of things. Although few inpatients will be receiving analytical psychotherapy, those who are may be seen by themselves and others as comprising an 'elitist group'. The fear that this may arouse feelings of jealousy in other patients or even the nurses should prove unfounded if the possibility is freely discussed at the appropriate meetings.

As we have seen, psychotherapy can be a traumatic experience for some patients and at times they will experience intense feelings of love or hatred towards their therapists. When this occurs, they may try to trick the nurse into confirming or denying their beliefs, and the nurse must take pains to avoid hinting at her opinion of the therapist.

Some patients may try to confide in a nurse, information which they say they cannot tell the therapist. This is a difficult situation and one that can usually be avoided if every patient is told on admission that it is a strict policy that there be no secrets. However, when it happens, it requires tactful handling. The nurse should tell the patient to discuss it with his therapist, or can offer to relay the message on his behalf. If this fails, the nurse may feel obliged to respect the patient's wishes unless she believes the information to indicate that his or someone else's life may be in danger. Then she must break the confidence.

Some patients may confide the same information to several members of staff, convincing them that they are the only ones to know. As they strive to protect the patient's interest, interstaff relationships may rapidly deteriorate, possibly exactly as he had planned.

Some forms of psychotherapy allow the nurse a more active part and this is particularly true of group psychotherapy. Many groups will have an experienced nurse as their leader or co-therapist and this is a challenging new experience.

Nurse learners may not graduate to group leadership but will be expected to participate. As a general rule they should be guided by the conduct of their more experienced colleagues, should avoid personal revelations or anecdotes, and should relax in the knowledge that they are unlikely to do lasting damage to their patients even if they do lack a certain finesse in group work. It is part of the leader's role to rescue the learner if the group should turn on her, making her the so-called scapegoat, or if she talks herself into a situation she cannot handle. An intense session of group psychotherapy can leave the participants drained and exhausted in a way that is less understandable than the tiredness generated on a busy surgical ward, but nevertheless, just as real.

Although unlikely during a short module, nurses with special aptitudes or enthusiasm may find themselves involved in supportive psychotherapy, in various behaviour modification programmes, or along with others in family or marital therapy.

To function adequately in any psychological form of treatment she will require a fair amount of self awareness and some idea of her own psychological blind spots. We would never dream of giving an injection without being familiar with a syringe. When our personality is the therapeutic tool of choice, ignorance can be just as inappropriate.

SUGGESTED READING

Barker P 1982 Behaviour therapy nursing. Croom Helm, London
Parry R 1983 Basic psychotherapy, 2nd edn. Churchill Livingstone, Edinburgh

8

The therapeutic community

We described in Chapter 3 the typical demeanour of a long-term psychiatric patient. We suggested that the apathy, submissiveness and total lack of self-direction seen in many such individuals are not symptoms specific to any one psychiatric illness and inferred that the treatment received in our hospitals was largely to blame for their present plight. It is rather ironic that the place where patients are sent to be treated can also be responsible for creating additional problems.

Goffman (1961) pointed out that psychiatric hospitals are not alone in producing these effects. Merchant ships, the Armed Forces, Prisoner of War Camps and various other establishments, being what he termed '*total institutions*', share many of their features.

In contrast to what is considered normal elsewhere, inmates of a total institution work, play, sleep and eat on the premises. All these activities are carried out, one after the other, in groups or batches under the auspices of a single authority. The system is rigidly hierarchical and the scope for individuality is strictly limited.

Besides fitting neatly into this model, the psychiatric hospital has also, through accident or design, become historically linked with the administrative philosophy of the general hospital.

Put somewhat simplistically, the traditional general hospital could be said to consist of three main groups of individuals: the doctor, the nurse and the patient.

The doctor

He (note always a man in the eyes of the public) is the glamour figure of the set-up. He makes the decisions, prescribes the treatment and expects to be obeyed. Because of his 'superior' training and intelligence, the public credit him with almost magical powers. He can make people better!

The nurse

She is definitely much further down the pecking order. The term is used by the public to describe both highly-trained and untrained individuals who attend to the patient's physical and biological needs. They carry out the doctor's instructions and may even make his coffee!

Like doctors, nurses tend to be idolised by the public and ascribed qualities that frankly they do not possess. Some patients, however, fantasise about the nurse's promiscuity and mythical sexual prowess.

The patient

Someone who is ill. He surrenders himself to the care of the others and is 'made better' by their skills. Consequently the patient is at the bottom of the pile!

While all hospitals obviously employ a large number of other people such as occupational therapists, porters, radiographers and cooks, each employee has a clearly-defined role. Everyone knows his place, everyone has a superior from whom to take orders and a subordinate to blame. This may sometimes be the patient.

Information and communication tend to flow from the top down and will be severely adulterated before reaching the patient. Messages directed upwards have to negotiate a large number of hurdles and are quite likely to get lost en route.

Although this is a blatant caricature, something vaguely similar may still have a place in the administration of a busy general hospital (on this the author feels unqualified to comment). However, more and more people would see it as entirely inappropriate for the care of the psychiatrically disordered.

The young mother of three pre-school children stuck in a multi-storey flat, the youth from an ethnic minority who has never been offered a job but who is periodically stopped and searched by the police for no good reason, or the spinster who has dedicated her life to the care of an increasingly ungrateful mother may all present quite genuinely as psychiatric patients. But it is ludicrous to assume that doctors and nurses operating traditionally can 'make them better'.

Irrespective of any heredity or constitutional disposition the examples highlighted clearly demonstrate areas of *social and interpersonal malfunctioning*. This is a common finding and even in situations where physical treatment can be very successful the majority of patients will require at least some help with interpersonal relationships. An approach which is based on unfettered communications and a close scrutiny of such relationships seems therefore to have a lot to offer.

Too often in the past, psychiatric hospitals have been filled with a large number of patients hoping to be seen by a tiny number of psychiatrists who, as likely as not, would have prescribed treatment that was empirical, or worse still, inappropriate. In the meantime, their care became custodial and completely alien to anything they would be likely to find in the world outside.

There is no such thing as a neutral environment. The sun shining through our bedroom window or the sound of a bird singing sets us up for the day, while burnt toast or a grumpy bus driver gets us off on the wrong foot. Our patients too are influenced by what goes on around them.

The ward and everything in it has great possibilities for therapeutic good or ill and in a therapeutic community the aim is to harness positively this potential.

This implies that every single aspect of the hospital's structure and function, as well as the behaviour and attitudes of every staff member, are crucial in determining the outcome of treatment. The patient population too has great therapeutic potential which is equally important and should be developed under staff supervision.

Therapeutic communities — a history

The dawn of the therapeutic community is traditionally considered to date from the Second World War and the immediate post-war period, although some people consider that the increased esteem in which the patient is held, had a parallel in the moral treatment of the 19th century.

During the Second World War there was a considerable amount of psychological disturbances amongst the troops, and few psychiatrists around to treat them. This led to the emergence of group therapies and the realisation that improvements could take place without the undivided, individual attention of a member of the medical staff. This encouraged the growth of the multidisciplinary approach to psychiatry.

In the subsequent post-war years socialist Britain set up the National Health Service. The mood in the country was such that the lot of the long-stay patients in run down hospitals began to prick a few consciences. An approach to care which gave patients a democratic involvement in their own treatment and offered hope of a substantial improvement in the quality of their life, seemed suited to the optimism of the time.

Dr Maxwell Jones emerged as a great innovator and the history of the therapeutic community is closely linked to his achievements. Jones developed his ideas while working with ex-prisoners of war in London. While initially his aim was to get his patients into groups so that he could teach them about various aspects of their condition, he found that by just listening to them, he learned a lot. By encouraging free communication and deliberately abdicating some of his autocratic powers, he allowed the patients to become active participants in their own treatment. Subsequently he established what was later to become the well-known Henderson Hospital.

From its beginning as a centre for the treatment of neurosis, it gradually evolved until it became a selective unit for the treatment of patients with psychopathic personalities. Patients were largely responsible for the day-to-day running of the unit and therapy was conducted through the daily community meetings and other small groups. Staff did not wear uniform and whatever their rank, were addressed by their Christian names. They came to be seen as enablers or facilitators rather than directors of treatment.

On his appointment as physician superintendent at Dingleton, a traditional mental hospital in the Scottish Border town of Melrose, Jones was able to develop his theories further. Eventually, the whole hospital was transformed into a therapeutic community and giant strides were made towards caring for a substantial proportion of the psychiatrically disturbed entirely outwith its gates.

Maxwell Jones and Dingleton Hospital gained inter-
national prominence in the 1960s and have greatly influenced the development of psychiatric care, both in the
UK and in the USA.

Jones's contribution took place at a time when
psychiatry generally was making rapid progress. The
liberating Mental Health Acts of 1959 (England and
Wales) and 1960 (Scotland) raised the status and esteem
of psychiatric patients. Following on the introduction of
new drugs, particularly the phenothiazines, these Acts
heralded an era of fresh hope.

The concept of the therapeutic community gained
rapid popularity in many quarters but also attracted a
good deal of criticism. Psychiatrists tended to split into
two camps: those who foresaw renewed hope in the
traditional methods, now reinforced by modern drugs
and ECT and those who favoured the more radical
approach advanced by Jones and his disciples. As the
predominant ideology in any hospital tends to be that of
the senior medical staff, it is harder for nurses to take a
lead in such matters, however many actively resisted the
changes which were necessary in setting up a therapeutic community.

Special features of a therapeutic community

The following represents a consensus of what makes up
the therapeutic community:

1. A flattening of the power hierarchy and a liberal
   sharing of leadership within the community.
2. Frequent face-to-face meetings of all regular
   members of the community.
3. All interpersonal tensions and conflicts dealt with
   by confrontation and working through, rather than
   by being repressed and treated as illness.
4. The fostering of a permissive but responsible
   environment.

We will consider these special features individually and in greater detail.

1. A flattening of the power hierarchy and a liberal sharing of leadership within the community

Frank, although still in his 30s, had been in hospital intermittently for many years. His serious psychiatric disorder was currently in remission and he displayed no florid symptoms.

A feature of Frank's condition, however, was his immaturity and periodic irresponsible behaviour. He might for instance leave the ward without telling anyone and return late for a meal, or shirk the ward duties which had been allocated to him. Going home for extended weekends was considered a crucial part of Frank's treatment, although his mother, with whom he lived, was elderly and slightly infirm. Since their home was 50 miles from the hospital, it was absolutely essential that he should behave responsibly during these visits.

After a few weeks, when Frank's behaviour had been mildly erratic, if unspectacular, he requested a weekend at home. The doctor's initial reaction was to turn him down flat. However, Frank disputed this at the next community meeting and following lengthy discussion the doctor was seen to be in the minority. In particular his fellow patients (who as a rule did not condone Frank's behaviour) and the more junior nursing staff (who saw most of him) felt he would be able to cope at home.

The decision was overturned.

Two points require further clarification:

a. In a traditional set-up the doctor would reach his decision, (hopefully after consultation with the nurse) and Frank would have no 'channels of appeal'. This would apply irrespective of how arbitrary or irrational it was or how lightly it had been taken.

b. The doctor did not grant the leave against his will because he had been outvoted. Rather, once he had been made aware of all the facts, he saw that his earlier opinion had been misguided.

This is important. The doctor cannot use the group's decision to opt out of his legal responsibility. In theory at least, he must retain the power of veto in the event of the group agreeing on a course of action which was obviously dangerous or illegal. Nevertheless, when a therapeutic community is functioning well this power of veto will normally lie dormant.

2. Frequent face-to-face meetings of all regular members of the community

This is a logical follow-on from the previous point. If democracy is to work and to be seen to work, regular meetings are essential. A main or 'community' meeting normally takes place daily, usually around 9.00 a.m. and is attended by everyone who is available. Other meetings with more selective functions may follow throughout the day.

Community meetings. The composition of this early morning group is interesting. It is not surprising that doctors and nurses of various grades should be expected to attend, while others such as occupational therapists, clinical psychologists and social workers also seem appropriate. However, some communities also expect the ward domestic, portering and gardening staff or tradesmen actively involved with the patients, to attend whenever possible. This is in keeping with the philosophy that everyone and everything in the patient's environment can directly influence his well-being.

The author once worked in a traditional psychiatric hospital where the consultant psychiatrist was astute, kindly and hard working. Sheer force of numbers, however, decreed that many of his long-term patients would only speak to him about once a year or less. Consequently his direct influence on the day-to-day quality of their life was minimal.

It was the brief misfortune of several patients to work

with a gardener, excellent at his job but totally unsuited to helping the psychiatrically disturbed. These patients spent several hours each day with the gardener and as a result were sometimes pretty miserable. Their daily peace of mind was chiefly influenced, not by the good quality of the medical staff but by the shortcomings of the ancillary worker — a vivid reminder of the importance of each member of the team.

When community meetings first take place, the topics discussed are usually rather mundane: the standard of food may be criticised or a patient may complain about his bath days or work schedules. Patients and staff may try to discuss a safe topic like holidays, thus effectively preventing other subjects, about which they feel anxious, being aired.

Only after it has become established that it is safe to criticise, that eccentricities will not be laughed at or that others may share an anxiety previously considered to be unique, will the barriers begin to drop and the real work start.

Eventually all happenings and emotions within the community will be analysed critically as they occur and lessons which may be learned from them, actively sought out.

Staff review meetings. These normally follow the community meeting with all staff attending. The accent is on informality and freedom in communication. Individual performances may come under scrutiny and staff members may be gently made aware of their own blind spots and prejudices.

Staff review meetings serve as an ideal training ground, perhaps giving the shy or reticent member a chance to practise speaking out before participating fully in the community meetings.

Patients' individual progress is also monitored during these sessions.

3. All interpersonal tensions and conflicts dealt with by confrontation and working through, rather than by being repressed and treated as a sign of illness

Traditionally if two psychiatric patients in a psychiatric hospital have a physical or violent verbal disagreement, they will be forcibly pulled apart and separated by the length of the ward. They may be given tranquillising drugs, they will certainly be told to see that it does not happen again and may be threatened with dire consequences if it does. Staff may consciously attempt to forget the incident and the issues leading up to it may be left unexplored. People living in close proximity cannot be kept apart for long, but while they are, old wounds may fester. When next they meet nothing will have changed and the risk of violence repeating itself is very great.

This approach to keeping the peace is exemplifed by the current trend of segregating rival soccer fans behind the netting wire, at different ends of the stadium. Lessons can be learned from the fact that this ploy is only partially successful. Violence at the match may be prevented but the dedicated hooligans can arrange to meet up in the streets or railway station and still give vent to their hostilities.

All of us can feel irritated or even angry with a colleague or patient. This may be rational — a colleague may continually arrive late, leaving us with an unfair burden — or irrational — a patient we like may respond much more favourably to someone else. What is clear is that while our irritation remains unvoiced, a tension will exist.

It is correctly said that an incohesive staff group will lead to a poorly functioning patient group. Inter-staff conflict can be sensed by the patients. They may feel themselves responsible or alternatively exploit it to their short-term advantage thus diverting attention from their own problems.

During the community meeting, therefore, it is considered essential that all interpersonal grievances are brought into the open where they may be used both as a learning tool and to encourage insight.

Crisis intervention groups. These take place immediately following an episode of violence, extreme verbal abuse or an attempt at self injury. All patients and staff who were involved or who chanced to be on the periphery meet under the chairmanship of a neutral individual to look at the incident. Factors leading up to it are explored, feelings discussed and a solution sought. This policy is in stark contrast to the 'segregate and sweep under the carpet' approach described above and has merit in its ability to prevent continual recurrences.

Staff sensitivity groups. Similarly, staff may meet on a regular, perhaps weekly, basis with the explicit purpose of looking at interpersonal feelings and tensions. Ideally this should reduce episodes of overt hostility and lead to less complicated interactions in the community meetings.

It can be uncomfortable to have your performances or even your personality commented on by your peers. Equally it may be difficult to discuss a colleague's negative attributes, particularly if you like them, or if they happen to be your superior. Only if an individual is safe in the knowledge that offence will not be taken at his well-meaning comments and that he will not subsequently be victimised, can such a group be successful. The problems encountered by nurses in such groups will be further discussed below.

Finally, in exploring attitudes and tensions within the community, we must resist the temptation to ascribe as 'mad' or 'sick' opinions or conduct of the patients in the group. Many ex-psychiatric patients, whose hospitalisation may have had nothing to do with their ability to reason adequately, complain that their friends and acquaintances no longer take them seriously in an argument, whatever the topic. If told a home truth we would rather deny, it is tempting to dismisss it as a symptom of the other's mental disorder. Such a blinkered attitude is unhelpful and completely contrary to the spirit of the therapeutic community.

The sponsoring of a permissive but responsible environment

This permissive aspect of the therapeutic community seems to be frequently misunderstood and is often seized on by detractors of the approach.

These criticisms may be fuelled by the occasional tendency towards 'acting out' by some patients or standards of cleanliness in the ward which would not be tolerated elsewhere. However, tales of permissiveness in the ordinary context of a laxity in attitudes to sex, violence and social deviancy seem to be grossly exaggerated and may give an interesting insight into the fantasy life of those who make the allegations.

Permissiveness as applied to a therapeutic community means the tolerating of deviant behaviour in as much as, once it has occurred, it is openly discussed rather than repressed by disciplinary action. Every member is encouraged to express himself honestly, without fear of punishment or ridicule. However, he is seen as being responsible for his own words and actions and anyone being deliberately obstructive or cruel would quickly be confronted with his behaviour. His need to indulge in such anti-group activities would be discussed and explored.

A much cited criticism of the permissive approach is that it is out of step with real life: that it is pointless providing a close, warm, accepting regime in hospital, when the world they hope to rejoin is often none of these things.

Paradoxically, however, it seems likely that unless an individual feels safe to express himself freely, he will not be able to experiment sufficiently to adapt to modern living.

Commonly encountered problems

A nurse new to the therapeutic community, particularly if she is also new to psychiatry, may feel vaguely 'for' its democratic principles but will be unsure of her own role in their implementation. She will not be alone!

While tradesmen, gardeners and other workers may have a lot to contribute, they are, after all, paid to do a job of work. Ward domestics are expected by their supervisors to keep the place clean, but cleaning up behind the patients can be seen as being anti-therapeutic.

Although junior members of staff may initially be over-whelmed by being included in the decision-making, *doctors and senior nurses* may have the most difficulty in readjusting. However keen they may be on the concept of power-sharing they are likely to find the sudden loss of their privileged status very harrowing at first. The charge nurse and ward sister, who once reigned supreme behind a row of badges and maybe even a frilly cap, will now have their decisions queried and their motives explored. Gone will be the day when their word was considered law, instead they will have to justify their courses of action. Worse, they will suddenly have to get used to being addressed as 'Doug' or 'Molly'. Some will adapt readily, others will take longer. Some may realistically decide that this is not for them and seek employment in a more traditional setting. This is preferable to their staying on, while passively resisting the ideals of the community.

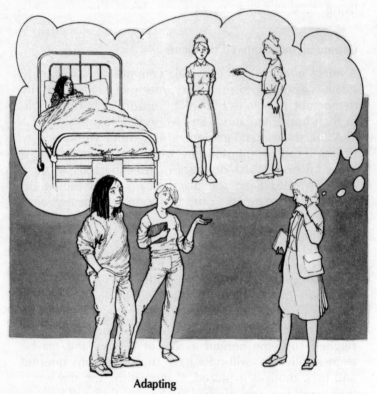

Adapting
to modern
trends

The young nurse will discover that a flattened hierarchy brings its own problems. She will, as part of the community, be party to the making of fairly far-reaching decisions and cannot shirk the responsibility this entails. At another level she may worry about her own contributions.

Does she speak enough? Does what she say make sense? Should she make what she considers to be a valid interjection when those around her, with much more experience, are saying nothing? How will she feel about being criticised by patients or by her colleagues? How close emotionally should she get to a patient?

She may wonder whether this dissolution of hierarchical authority rings entirely true. While it is all right to question Doug or Molly's attitudes during a meeting, they will eventually write the assessment on which the nurse's progress in training will partially depend.

The wide demands of general nurse training mean that the student nurse cannot hope to be totally assimilated into the therapeutic community, but those who are impressed may return to do their psychiatric training and to specialise.

Areas of competence

The therapeutic community is tried and tested in the rehabilitative treatment of long-term psychiatric patients, it is a commonly-used approach in acute admission areas and Henderson Hospital set a precedent for the care of those with personality disorders. Alcoholics, drug addicts and individuals diagnosed as having psychopathic personalities seem attracted to its principles and it is also widely used amongst self-help and voluntary caring organisations.

In Barlinnie Prison, Scotland in 1973, an exciting experiment took place. Some of the most violent prisoners, who because of their records, had until then been locked up in harsh and repressive circumstances, were introduced to the 'special unit'.

The unit is run on the basis of a therapeutic community and incorporates a degree of democracy and informality, previously unheard of in a penal institution. Despite considerable resistance from the more traditional prison officers and some sections of the media, the results, although inconclusive, have been promising. Prison violence and serious assaults on prison officers have fallen dramatically.

The future

The therapeutic community may have lost some of the radical, trail-blazing appeal which characterised it in the 1960s. Some would say it has passed its peak of popularity and usefulness but this is debatable.

Although large scale adoption of its ideals (as happened at Dingleton) no longer takes place, its principles have been widely accepted in a more modified form.

The concepts of patient involvement, confrontation and the right of everyone to have his voice heard are the very essence of the therapeutic community. They are no longer considered controversial and have permeated vast areas of once traditional psychiatric care.

REFERENCE

Goffman E 1961 Asylums: essays on the social situation of mental patients and other inmates. Penguin, Harmondsworth.

SUGGESTED READING

Boyle J 1977 A sense of freedom. Canongate, Edinburgh
Janson E (ed) 1980 The therapeutic community. Croom Helm, London

PART | THREE

PSYCHIATRY
MADE SIMPLE

Sigmund Freud (1856–1939)
Oral, anal and phallic stages of development
Id, ego and superego
Mental defence mechanisms
Some criticisms
Modern life and mental health

9

The development of the personality

Anyone who has seen a newborn baby, helpless and neurologically immature, must marvel at the process which eventually transforms it into a fully functioning adult. The physical maturation, although obvious and great, may be less than the psychological changes that occur. As far as we can determine the human species alone has the capacity to experience emotions such as guilt, or the ability to foresee the possible consequences of any course of action on which it might embark. These develop gradually as the years slip by and the child struggles towards adulthood. In every case the end result will be a unique individual with his own inimitable personality.

The thinking nurse will realise that the factors influencing personality development are many, complicated and largely immeasurable. She should not be surprised, therefore, to learn that thoughts on the subject tend to be hypothetical rather than indisputable facts. Equally, she will discover that no one theory pleases everyone, and that many different 'schools' exist, all with their own ideas and emphasis.

This chapter seeks merely to introduce the nurse

learner to the concept of personality development, in order to allow some understanding of what may previously have been unfathomable aspects of the patients in her care. It is based mainly on Freudian theory, although other viewpoints are considered in the final chapter of the book.

Sigmund Freud (1856–1939), although originally a neurologist, carried out exhaustive studies on large numbers of individuals, observing them closely and recording meticulously, all he thought he saw. His ideas were controversial, but represented a giant step forward in the understanding of the human personality.

The acknowledgement of the existence of the 'unconscious' (Ch. I) is crucial in the understanding of Freud, as is the acceptance of the idea of repression. This is the individual's ability to relegate unknowingly to his unconscious, vast amounts of material which are thereby completely 'forgotten'. Such concepts are now widely accepted.

The human baby is born in an immature state, with a set of basic, if keenly felt, biological needs. As parents everywhere can testify, the infant cannot postpone gratification of any of those needs and as a result, will yell ferociously for a drink at 2 a.m. or defecate unconcernedly on mother's best dress, the living room carpet or the family's precious christening shawl.

During this stage the infant is said to conduct himself purely in accordance with the 'pleasure principle'. In his continued maturation the role of mother or a substitute is absolutely vital.

Slowly he must come to realise that he is not the centre of the universe. The realisation that mother is not merely a tap that can be turned on to satisfy his biological cravings for food, warmth and affection may arouse feelings of anger or distress. This hitherto entirely positive regard for mother who was literally his lifeline, may now be tempered with feelings of hate. How dare she deny him his pleasures? When feelings of love and hate occur at the same time, this is called *ambivalence*.

At this stage all the baby's sensations of pleasure arrive via the mouth. We do not know the emotions a distraught infant is experiencing, but can readily see how he will relax as soon as he is put to the breast or given a bottle. Important though the taking of nourishment is, it is not the sole function of the mouth. Thumb sucking and the use of a commercial comforter — 'the dummy' — are widespread, yet if all that was desired was food, they would be rapidly discarded on the realisation that it was not forthcoming. That they are not, appears to suggest that these oral activities are a source of pleasure, comfort or security in their own right. As he gets a little older, the infant quickly sets about exploring his immediate environment — by sticking it in his mouth! With enviable dexterity he will locate and subsequently suck his toes while rattles, teddy bears and his cot side will all be given the same treatment during this period of intense discovery.

Because of the importance of the mouth during this time, the period from birth to around 15 months is termed the *oral* phase of development. Some examples of oral behaviour such as smoking, pencil chewing or eating for comfort may be exhibited by some individuals throughout their life without causing undue comment.

Gradually the child will develop the capacity to postpone his immediate desires. He will come to realise that mother is not around all the time and that he must wait for his meals. As toilet-training begins, he will discover that indiscriminate soiling will no longer be tolerated and eventually he will come to terms with the need to use a potty or toilet at an appropriate time. He is now beginning to function according to the *reality principle*.

At this stage the infant will be intensely aware of and increasingly interested in his excretory functions. The feelings of embarrassment or disgust attributed by many

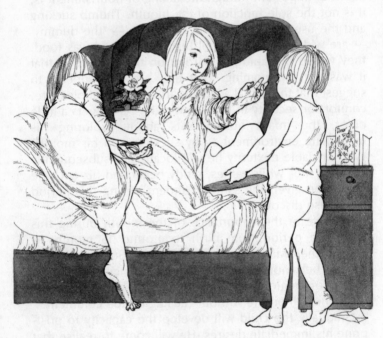

**CONDUCT
UNBECOMING!**

adults to the act of defecation are conspicuously absent. The toddler will show off his faeces with the unqualified pride appropriate to this, the first thing he has produced unaided! The passing of faeces is experienced as a pleasurable sensation and it must come as a great disappointment to the youngster to discover that society, in the shape of mother, imposes strict rules as to when and where such conduct is permissible.

Toilet-training may produce a tremendous battle of wills before the infant proves ready to relinquish the pleasure of unbridled excretion, in order to conform to mother's wishes. A child who is uncertain of mother's unconditional love, or who is forced to commence training while neurologically unready may have great difficulty at this time. The need to establish a routine and deposit the faeces appropriately can have a lasting effect on some adults who develop a rigid unbending personality and an obsessional desire for neatness or precision.

Because of the importance of excretion and the excretory organs during this phase, the period from approximately 15 months to 3 or 4 years is termed the *anal* phase of development.

By the time the child reaches this age, a subtle change will have occurred in the previously all-encompassing relationship with mother. Perhaps a brother or sister will have been born to demand a share of mother's time and affections, but in any case, other people will be becoming increasingly significant.

Father, during the first year of his child's life, is frequently described as being a 'shadowy' figure, languishing somewhere in the periphery of his experience. This perhaps does less than justice to the large number of fathers who are closely involved from the start, and ignores completely the significant number who may never be around at all.

Nevertheless, the child will become increasingly aware of and involved with his father. He will be intrigued with the special, but not fully understood relationship shared by his parents. Children will become intensely interested in the anatomical differences between the sexes and in the appearance of their own bodies. Because the chief area of interest and pleasure has now switched to the genitalia, this period is called the *phallic* stage of development. (Phallus is another name for penis, the male sexual organ.)

At this stage the small girl, on seeing her naked brother, may feel that her penis has somehow been removed. The young boy may fear that his, too, may be cut off if he does something wrong — a situation known as *castration anxiety*.

The author, while relaxing by a duck pond with his family, once overheard an elderly lady threaten her small grandson standing too near the edge that a fish would jump out and bite off his 'willie'. Nonsensical as such a notion seems to a mature adult, coming from a supposedly wise grandparent it must have appeared a frightening possibility. The youngster jumped back to safety, but the cost to his psychological equilibrium can only be guessed at!

With an awareness of genital pleasure comes a wish to share it with the significant others in their life. For the small boy, this means his mother. However, he perceives such desires as dangerous. He may feel in competition with father for mother's affections, and may wish to take his place. Nevertheless, he loves his father and is impressed by his size. He is a formidable rival.

Likewise, the small girl will openly compete with mother for her father's attentions, but will again be anxious that her feelings may result in punishment.

This complicated state of affairs, Freud called the *Oedipal conflict*. (Oedipus was a prince in Greek mythology, who, separated from his parents at an early age, unknowingly slew his father in battle and married his mother.) Freud had an interesting, if eccentric, habit of using mythology to illustrate many of his theories.

Unresolved conflicts from this stage of development are frequently cited as being responsible for subsequent psychiatric disorder. Indeed children who are punished or, perhaps more commonly, ridiculed for trying to come to terms with these vaguely felt emotions, may in adulthood be unable to express themselves sexually, or give of themselves in a mature way, since they have learned that to do so, leaves them vulnerable and exposed.

Some adults will tremble with trepidation in the presence of authority figures, largely because they have never come to terms with this original rival situation, when the odds were so obviously stacked against them. Nurses, in the hierarchical structure in which they are employed, may find themselves feeling like this, but also, particularly on becoming qualified, may be attributed parental qualities by some of their patients.

Some ward sisters appear unconsciously to see the consultant as a father figure. They may, on the one hand, be flirtatious or familiar, aware of the special relationship which in reality they have with him. At the same time, however, they may hold him in exaggerated awe, with his word being very much law. Such daily happenings can be seen as a re-enactment of the earlier, perhaps inadequately dealt with, Oedipal conflicts. The same applies to the possibly more serious situation of a young person, usually female, embarking on an affair or marriage with someone many years her senior.

The few short years from birth till about 6 years of age as discussed above are hectic as far as personality development is concerned. They are followed however by a period of relative calm, known as the years of *latency*. This takes the individual up to the turbulent years of adolescence which are usually traumatic, and which for some may even herald a psychiatric breakdown.

It is difficult to accept all the foregoing material as fact, and many nurses may be incredulous or may angrily deny that they were ever party to such nonsense. This argument can be countered by pointing to the mechanism of repression.

Maturing through the developmental stages is far from uncomplicated and in some cases will have been positively painful. Mercifully most of our psychological growing pains are removed from our awareness and remain buried, often forever, in our unconscious.

ID, EGO AND SUPEREGO

The mind for convenience sake is often described as being split into three components the id, the ego and the superego. It must be stressed that this is a functional rather than a physical differentiation and these parts cannot be demonstrated, dissected or drawn.

The most basic level of function, concerned with the primitive, biological needs and governed by the pleasure principle is present from birth and is called the *id*. It is totally self-centred and the focus of all primary desire. It demands instant and total satisfaction and takes no account of reality.

With the development of the *ego* a more mature pattern of behaviour is seen. The infant learns to postpone id urges. It comes to realise that mother cannot always be around and furthermore, if she is summoned too often, her approach will be less tender and the experience will be spoiled. Behaviour now takes into account the demands of real life and the cravings of the id will frequently be thwarted. This stage of development is governed by the reality principle.

Even now, although the individual may be able to guess at the possible outcome of any piece of behaviour, an inner sense of rightness or wrongness will be totally absent. This arrives only with the development of the *superego* which corresponds roughly to the lay term 'conscience' and produces internal checks on behaviour, which if ignored, cause the individual to experience feelings of guilt.

The superego does not develop until around the age of 6 or 7 years and varies greatly in its degree of 'strictness'. A middle-aged lady of the author's acquaintance feels overwhelmingly guilty should she wash her clothes on a Sunday, while several convicted murderers, whom he has known professionally, show no remorse when discussing their sometimes heinous offences.

Roughly the individual adopts similar standards to those of his parents, so that a child brought up in a family where stealing is condoned will not feel guilty when he does likewise. A youngster, who as his superego is developing, has only unsuitable models to copy, or perhaps as in the case of a boy from a one parent family, no model of the same sex, will be at a disadvantage. This could result in his moral standards being well outside the 'normal' range.

Id, ego and superego — an everyday example

A married man at a party is extremely attracted to a young woman who, it transpires, is the wife of his employer. His id would 'urge' him to approach her, with a view to persuading her to make love. A basic instinct (sex) has been aroused, and should be gratified to the exclusion of all else.

The ego would immediately disagree. The reality of the situation suggests such action would be ill-advised. What about his wife? How would she react?

His boss would probably sack him, and might even thump him on the jaw. The possible consequences would seem to outweigh the momentary joy of the flesh.

The question of consequences would be entirely irrelevant to the superego. For some people, 'Thou shalt not commit adultery' is an unnegotiable rule. No proposition would be made because the man, entirely within himself, feels that to do so, would be morally wrong.

This simplistic example erroneously conjures up a picture of an individual being continuously faced with a battery of options, from which he can make a rational choice. While at the party in question the man may just have been aware of the various possibilities listed, in reality our confrontations usually take place at an unconscious level.

Ideally, the various aspects of the personality should be smoothly interrelated; the mature or so-called 'well-balanced' individual conducts his life in such a way that the conflicting demands of his instincts, the real live world, and his own moral standards are seldom consciously recognised.

A feeling of anxiety is the outward signal that this psychological synchronisation is threatening to break down. Being anxious involves a feeling of apprehension which may lead to a state of tension, although the cause of this disquiet may not be recognised.

Anxiety can be perfectly natural and functional. We may be anxious about failing examinations, so we study hard, or we adopt more healthy eating habits as a result of anxiety about our well-being.

On the other hand, anxiety may arise as a result of instinctual pressure from the id. In particular, many people are unconsciously afraid that they may be unable to control their aggressive or sexual impulses and may become anxious in situations such as parties or arguments, when this seems likely to be put to the test.

Finally there is moral anxiety or guilt, which may arise from offending the super ego or breaking our individually set code of conduct.

Anxiety in its most severe form may appear as a frank psychiatric disorder, either diffusely spread around, or focused on a particular situation, — the phobia. Moreover, many other psychiatric conditions are frequently explained as being a maladaptive attempt to cope with anxiety.

Some nurses will agree that they feel anxious from time to time, but may claim that the reason for this is usually obvious. They may deny that they wander around full of festering conflicts and may suggest that we have overstated the importance of anxiety.

This argument overlooks the individual's self-correcting devices which are continually striving to maintain the psychological equilibrium. These are called mental defence mechanisms and are used to some extent by us all as we unconsciously strive to ward off anxiety.

MENTAL DEFENCE MECHANISMS

Repression

This is perhaps the most basic of all defence mechanisms. It describes the transferring of thoughts, memories and emotions from conscious awareness to the unconscious. The extent to which any individual uses repression is impossible to demonstrate (the evidence is lost in the unconscious), but it seems likely that we all protect our self image by banishing unacceptable parts of our self from our awareness.

We do not remember the traumas of early childhood. We cannot recall the ambivalence we felt towards our mother who protected us, but who gradually denied us the gratification of our every whim, or the struggle of wills involved in toilet-training. When we first hear of the concept of the Oedipal complex we may greet it with scepticism, humour or angry denial. This reaction could be due to the fact that the idea is genuinely absurd, but conversely our incongruity could arise because all the relevant material has been repressed.

Many of the principles of modern psychotherapy involve this repressed material. One school of thought suggests mental illness arises as a result of vaguely felt repressions striving to re-establish themselves on the surface.

Repressed material may find expression during our dreams, in acute and severe episodes of mental disorder, or as a result of therapy.

Denial

That which is threatening or unacceptable merely ceases to exist for the individual using denial. Children are adept at employing this mechanism which is also so common as to be considered a normal stage of bereavement. The new widow will tell the policeman at her door that he is mistaken. Her husband was perfectly normal this morning and the victim of the road accident is obviously someone else. Denial is not a conscious mechanism, even although it may be obvious to everyone but the person using it.

> John was 42 years old and above average intelligence. He had seen his father and uncle die with the distressing hereditary condition of Huntington's chorea, which is known to affect 50 % of a sufferer's offspring. It commonly manifests itself in the 30s or 40s. In conversation with the author, John, who was seeking advice on some other pretext was seen to exhibit marked jerking movements of the face and arms. He spoke reasonably about his problems of being part of a family cursed with Huntington's chorea, but seemed convincing when he asserted, 'Thankfully, I seem to have missed it'.

Denial of a similar but less dramatic quality is frequently seen in general hospitals. Patients who may be seriously ill, or about to undergo a dangerous operation may appear genuinely jovial or carefree. On such occasions it may be good nursing practise to leave well alone although it is important to be able to differentiate between these patients and others who may merely be putting on an act. The latter group may benefit from active counselling.

Rationalisation

Here the individual offers a plausible and indeed usually noble reason for a piece of behaviour or course of action.

If we support a soccer team who are failing to win any matches, we may say that it is because they concentrate too much on skilful or attacking play and do not bend the rules or kick their opponents to the same extent as do other teams.

Senior Nurses who interview would-be entrants to the profession will be familiar with the usual answers given to the age-old question, 'Why do you want to become a nurse?'

Invariably, we are told of her desire to help people less well off than herself, of a wish to repay the service for a period of past hospitalisation, or of her great love for children, the elderly or the mentally handicapped. Many youngsters will wish to nurse for just those reasons, but for others it will be something entirely different. We seldom hear of the fact that nursing is a secure job, (relatively), that the hospital is just around the corner, or that she fancies having the occasional morning free to drink coffee or go window shopping. She may be too dim to be a dentist, too ugly to be a model or too poor to drive racing cars. Yet we hear only the acceptable repetitions.

Rationalisation is widely used and helps maintain our feelings of worthiness. Nevertheless, individuals who employ this device excessively seem dangerously out of touch with reality.

Sublimation

This allows potentially anti-social drives, usually of an aggressive or sexual nature, to find expression in an acceptable form. Often quoted is the example of the young man who channels his aggression towards sport rather than becoming overtly violent.

Society and his individual conscience may condone 'healthy competitiveness' in a rugby scrum but will rightly object to a telephone kiosk being vandalised. It is interesting to note that many of the world's greatest artistic achievements are the work of homosexuals who lived usually at a time when direct expression of homosexuality was much less acceptable than it is today.

Women, who by some quirk of fortune are denied the experience of motherhood, may dedicate their lives to nursing or to looking after other people's children. Although this is frequently given as an example of sublimation it is an inaccurate description. Their drives are not of an anti-social nature and therefore do not require to be altered. Their so-called 'maternal instincts' achieve direct gratification, albeit with someone other than their natural offspring. This could more accurately be called *substitution*.

Conversion

This is the hysteria which seemed to be so familiar to Freud and others of that era. Here the inner tensions and conflicts are replaced by a bodily symptom, which however has no physical cause.

Sometimes, as in the case of the student who develops a paralysis of the right hand prior to an examination, it seems obvious that the symptoms somehow protect the patient. Martin's knee injury (Ch. 7) would possibly belong to this category. Nevertheless, it is important to realise that the patient with a conversion symptom is not malingering and that the condition is very real to him. Nor is it easy to know for certain when a symptom has a physical basis. A paralysed limb may be the result of conversion, but could be caused by a brain tumour!

The symptoms associated with conversion can sometimes be successfully removed by hypnosis or some form of behaviour therapy, but great caution is required. By removing the symptoms without in any way explaining or altering the original cause of the anxiety, the therapist may merely be kicking away the patient's psychological crutch. Similar, or completely different, symptoms may therefore appear.

Reaction formation

This may be considered a more permanent mechanism, by which forbidden desires or personality features are replaced by others which are the exact opposite. Thus someone with strong, unconscious aggressive tendencies may present as a pacifist, while others who parade their moral righteousness for all to see, may harbour deep rooted sexual fantasies or desires.

The true nature of these personalities may partially reveal themselves in dreams, psychiatric disorder or during periods of extreme stress. Perhaps this is the mechanism that allows supposedly devout Christians to lead the clamour for the restoration of hanging, and meek old ladies to attack wrestlers with umbrellas or hat pins.

Displacement

Here pent-up emotions or fears are redirected from their primary source to another which may be reviewed with more social approval.

A young man, unconsciously afraid of having contracted venereal disease, may present with a fear of cancer, or a woman frightened by her vaguely felt promiscuous desires may develop agrophobia, a fear of open spaces. In hospital, at least some of the complaints about the food may be a manifestation of displacement.

Somehow it is easier to complain of a sausage than a surgeon!

This mechanism is probably behind the formation of many apparently irrational phobias and supports the argument against removing symptoms without exploring their cause.

Projection

This allows the individual to disown unconsciously unacceptable parts of himself and attribute them to someone else.

An old Yiddish proverb says 'The girl who can't dance, says the band can't play,' while we are all familiar with the bad workman who blames his tools.

A husband who wishes to avoid sexual relationships with his wife may accuse her of frigidity, while one who has been unfaithful may unconsciously distort the facts to convince himself that his wife has been unfaithful to him. In world politics, the great powers continually accuse each other of spying, naked aggression and abuse of human rights, even though evidence points to the fact that they too are directly involved in just those activities. In the wards, a patient who is openly suspicious or who blames other patients or nurses for their callousness, sloth or immorality may be using projection to fend off the recognition of those very characteristics in himself.

Introjection

This is almost the exact opposite of projection, and involves the turning inwards of emotions or drives which should more healthily be expressed.

A wife widowed at an early age could justifiably feel, amongst other things, a sense of anger at her husband for leaving her to cope on her own. Of course it is unlikely that she could express this or even recognise it, but such feelings can adversely affect her ability to resolve her natural grief. Interestingly, on such occasions, the wife may unwittingly adopt certain characteristics or mannerisms of her husband and may find herself reacting to situations in a way typical of him.

Introjection can sometimes play an important part in the formation of depression with the victim attributing to himself all the wickedness, corruption and vice which may more accurately be seen to belong to the world about him. In an effort to atone, or merely to exterminate the evil of which he is so acutely aware, suicide or self injury may be contemplated and may be carried out with some determination.

Regression

This is quite often seen by nurses. It involves the individual, under stress, reverting to behaviour more suitable to an earlier period in his development. Classically, it appears in the young child who may feel replaced in his parents' affections on the arrival of a new brother or sister. Such children, although possibly appearing to love the baby, may suddenly revert to soiling or wetting themselves, or to talking in a baby voice. It seems as if they are unconsciously attempting to recapture a time when life was less stressful.

Some psychiatric patients may regress to quite an immature level during their illness, while others will appear to get stuck at one level and never mature beyond it. This is called *fixation*.

In a general ward, where realistic anxiety and enforced dependency go hand in hand, regression can often be spotted. Patients may compete with one another for the nurse's attentions or sulk over trivial incidents. The patient who, on seeing someone else being given a bed pan, immediately requests one for himself, may be re-enacting the sibling rivalry of his childhood.

Finally, nurses too, can regress. The author, in the College of Nursing where he is employed, has during particularly stressful parts of the course, witnessed several learners, busily sucking their thumbs!

The above are only a few of the more common mental defence mechanisms used by countless individuals in their daily life. The nurse must realise that the patient has no idea as to why he is behaving as he is and moreover will be unaware that his actions are anything other than straightforward.

The defence mechanism of *suppression* is somewhat different. Here the individual makes a conscious and deliberate effort to put something to the back of his mind. Most of us will use this technique from time to time and be aware of its limitations. The very effort of planning to 'forget' the implication of a forthcoming examination, or the fact that we have to get up early the morning after a party tends to focus our attention towards it, thus achieving the exact opposite of the desired effect.

Spotting defence mechanisms can be largely an intellectual and pointless exercise if practised on the population at large. Unfortunately, many readers may come across colleagues in pubs or at parties who delight in loudly exposing the mental defence mechanisms used by others in their company. Usually they are insensitive bores with only an elementary knowledge of psychiatry. Perhaps they should examine their own need to act so smart.

One of the reasons why nurses training for the general register are required to have psychiatric experience is so that they will be better able to meet the needs of all their patients by deepening their knowledge of psychological matters. Merely being able to spot mental defence mechanisms is of limited value. The perceptive nurse will realise that the need to employ such devices is indicative of underlying anxiety and will strive to understand and alleviate it.

Our view of personality development — some criticisms

Any theory which attempts to explain tritely something as complicated as the development of human personality in a few short paragraphs, must be open to criticism. Such a theory is likely to be oversimplified and full of generalisations.

It has been pointed out that Freud's patients were largely middle-aged, middle class European females, suffering from hysteria and living in some cases during the reign of Queen Victoria.

Can his theories be carried forward a century and applied uncritically to the alcoholic offshore worker, the culture shocked, non-English speaking immigrant or the unemployed tenant of a decaying, high rise flat? We will see how some of Freud's professional disciples split with him to form their own schools of psychology.

One such former orthodox Freudian psychoanalyst was Karen Horney. Her contribution is largely concerned with the effect of the environment on the personality. Freud saw the environment as being a distillation of the individuals who make it up. It could be changed only if these individuals changed.

Horney and her followers adopted the opposite view. They regarded individuals as being moulded by the culture of which they are members. If the environment could be altered, they too would change.

Horney had practised in Germany before escaping to the USA during the ascendancy of the Nazis in the 1930s and it is interesting to postulate as to how she personally had changed in these contrasting cultures. Like Freud she believed that early life experiences largely influence the shape of the adult personality, but she believed this personality remains flexible. In response to environmental factors it can continue to develop throughout life.

This is possibly more optimistic from a therapeutic point of view. It implies that things like government intervention in poor housing areas, education, or personal endeavour could influence favourably the mental health of large numbers of individuals. Although a tall order, it is more attainable than psychoanalysis for the masses.

MODERN LIFE AND MENTAL HEALTH

Let us agree in the meantime with the description in this chapter of how the child's personality develops in its early years. After all, a considerable amount of it is based on observable and observed material. Unfortunately, it presupposes an ideal situation.

Mother is loving, food is available and father, although 'shadowy', is around. Presumably he leaves for work each morning after kissing everyone goodbye, only to return promptly in the evening having earned sufficient money to meet the family's needs. He and he alone shares mother's bed.

Such a set-up may have been universal at some point in history (although there are good reasons to doubt it) but it no longer applies to a significant proportion of the population.

Divorce is said to be the outcome of one marriage in three and the trend continues upwards. While this may reduce the long-term trauma of children being brought up in a loveless environment, divorces take time. Young children may be deprived of a suitable same sex model at a vital period in their upbringing. They may be asked to change models on the remarriage of the parent with whom they live, or may suddenly discover a number of short-term adults briefly 'passing through' as the parent struggles to adjust to the marriageless state. A child, who during the Oedipal stage of development suddenly discovers that the rival parent has left for good, may blame himself, and develop an irrational fear of his destructive capabilities. An alarming aspect of this is the fact that there appears to be some connection between rejection in childhood and the later development of the extremely serious personality disorder, psychopathy.

One-parent families have much in common with this group since many single parents are in fact divorcees. However, despite the availability of almost fool-proof contraception, illegitimacy remains with us. Although the stigma of unmarried parenthood has diminished, (more single females nowadays may in fact choose to become pregnant) illegitimacy still has important implications for the child. Moral issues apart, the problem of finding a suitable same sex model is also applicable to this group.

Moreover, it has been established that single-parent families are often closely linked with *poverty*. In the UK single parents are entitled to a small additional allowance from the State but this is insufficient to pay for child-minders or to improve substantially the standard of living.

Poverty is also closely linked with **unemployment**, which seems set to become a permanent feature of modern living. Adolescents may come from a home where the adults have seldom been able to find work. They in turn may leave school with little chance of ever working and even less of finding a job suited to their needs and aptitudes. The implication of prolonged, enforced inactivity on the mental health of such individuals gives rise to growing concern.

Another feature in many parts of today's society is the presence of **ethnic minority groups**. Some ethnic groups assimilate into the cultural pattern of the host country very easily, while others stick rigidly to what is familiar.

Children of ethnic minorities may go to school with children from a variety of cultures, many of whom will question or even ridicule the previously considered sacrosanct values of the home. Attitudes to religion, the role of women, parental authority or fixed marriages may be actively challenged by the younger generation, much to the anger, dismay and bewilderment of the adults.

Prejudice is an ugly aspect of multiracial living and although it is often subjective, its presence is keenly felt by many families of non-European origins. Long-term subjection to prejudices must have a detrimental effect on the psychological well-being and self-esteem of its victims.

Nurses, themselves recruited from ethnic minorities, can be invaluable in ensuring that these groups avail themselves of the facilities on offer, since some beliefs, customs and norms will seem inexplicable to others charged with their care. The forging of close links with each minority's community leaders and representatives is a priority, especially when such nurses are not available.

Children born into the latter part of the 20th century are bombarded with a barrage of stimuli that could never have been anticipated 100 years ago. Almost immediately the life-sustaining mother and shadowy dad will be in competition for the infant's attention with teeming motorways, flashing neon lights and the magic box in the corner.

The influence of **television** on the development of the child's personality cannot be demonstrated, but must be considerable. On the one hand, from an early age he can watch live before breakfast, events in some far corner of the globe. At a similar age, his grandparents would not have known such places existed! The more formal educational programmes for infants upwards are usually excellent.

On the other hand, very young children can witness

scenes of unbelievable violence literally every day of their lives. They learn to laugh at cartoons depicting cats being forced through mincing machines or flattened by heavy hammers, while killings in television dramas, unless particularly spectacular, hardly merit a second glance.

Television can go a long way towards filling a vacuum by providing suitable models for children who may be denied them in the flesh. For many children, a newscaster or presenter of a Saturday morning television show may be more familiar than their own father!

The possiblity that it does just the opposite and provides unsuitable examples is extremely worrying. The influence of television on personality development is not clear cut but could be considerable. It deserves to be taken seriously and further evaluated.

Conclusion

Society, and the people who comprise it, have changed radically since Freud first produced his writings. Nevertheless his description of the newborn's tortuous progress towards adulthood provides considerable insight into the workings of the mind and the possible development of psychiatric disorder. Environmental factors are many and different and obviously influential. Their contribution should not be minimised.

SUGGESTED READING

Brown J A C 1961 Freud and the post Freudians. Penguin, Harmondsworth

Burns R B 1980 Essential psychology. MTP Press, Lancaster

Maddison D, Kellehear K J 1982 Psychiatric nursing, 5th edn. Churchill Livingstone, Edinburgh

Mangen S P 1982 Sociology and mental health. Churchill Livingstone, Edinburgh

Parry R 1983 Basic psychotherapy, 2nd edn, Churchill Livingstone, Edinburgh

10

A classification of psychiatric illness

WHY CLASSIFY?

Some readers may be surprised to find a classification of psychiatric illness in a book specifically written for nurses. Radical individuals may deny the very existence of psychiatric illness, while others suggest that giving people labels is seldom helpful.

It is the author's frequently stated belief that everyone, whether a psychiatric patient or not, is very much an individual and he deplores any attempt at pigeon-holing people into narrow diagnostic categories. It would be possible to describe the problems and nursing requirements of all our patients using a simple non-medical vocabulary. It would also be so cumbersome as to be bordering on the ridiculous.

People who come, or are brought to a psychiatric hospital for treatment, tend to exhibit their signs and symptoms in one of several clearly recognisable clusters. They are therefore usually given a diagnosis.

Problems of classification

Often medical conditions are classified according to their cause, but this does not work in psychiatry. Too often the causes of any condition are diffuse, and are usually unknown. This means that psychiatric classifications are often seen as being less satisfactory usually being entirely descriptive, e.g. 'depression' or 'anxiety'. The danger in such classifications is that they tend to create the impression that a label, once applied becomes a concrete entity, e.g. 'schizophrenia', when all it can really do is describe a recognisable cluster of signs and symptoms. Although imprecise, classification is nevertheless generally considered to be useful.

Table 10.1 is not copied slavishly from any particular learned document, but should be familiar to many psychiatric workers. It sees as important the initial recognition and separation of *psychosis and neurosis*.

Psychosis is a serious form of mental disorder, usually severe enough to involve a grave disorganisation of the personality associated with a disturbed perception of reality. Consequently, symptoms such as delusions or hallucinations can be present, but insight may be missing.

This means that the non-psychiatrically disturbed person may have difficulty in 'putting themselves in such a person's shoes,' and is unlikely to appreciate fully what he is going through. Psychosis may be subdivided into 'organic' or 'functional', depending on whether or not a demonstrable change (as in dementia) has occurred within the brain.

Neurosis represents an abnormal emotional reaction to stress which tends to block or inhibit the individual's talents and instincts. Neurosis is the most common faulty response to life's stresses and may manifest itself in varying degrees.

The individual remains in touch with reality, may realise that something is wrong and will not experience hallucinations or delusions.

It is sometimes said that everyone is neurotic to some extent and at least it is easier for most people to empathise with this type of malfunctioning.

Personality disorders which are sometimes called character neuroses cannot confidently be ascribed the label, mental illness. Instead they represent often deeply ingrained traits or typical responses which are sufficiently removed from the average to be classed 'abnormal'. As these traits are usually well-established they may be accepted by the individual and others as being 'part' of himself and are therefore likely to be resistive to attempts at change.

Psychosomatic disorders I have considered as a separate category. They are physical illnesses or symptoms for which emotional factors are responsible or to which they contribute significantly.

It is important to appreciate that genuine, demonstrable signs and symptoms are present (e.g. a duodenal ulcer) but that these have been exacerbated by stress. It is impossible to state with any certainty which conditions are psychosomatic in origin, although ulcers, asthma and various skin complaints are generally accepted as being good examples. Some people believe that a wide variety of illnesses are psychosomatic and would definitely include myocardial infarction (heart attack) and even some forms of carcinoma in their list. Anorexia nervosa discussed in Chapter 16 is a condition which is difficult to categorise, but it too is often classed as psychosomatic.

It is important to realise that even when an emotional link can be established, the sufferer cannot be expected to 'will' away the symptoms. He therefore deserves the same sympathetic approach afforded to other patients.

Table 10.1 represents a workable attempt at classifi-

Table 10.1 A classification of psychiatric illness

Psychosis		Neurosis	Personality Disorders
Organic	Functional	Abnormal Emotional Reactions (symptom neuroses)	(character neuroses)
1. Acute (reversible) Delirium, confused states	1. Affective disorders (Mood)	1. Anxiety state	Schizoid*
Examples Delirium, confused drug intoxication	a. Mania/hypomania	2. Phobic state	Cyclothymic*
	b. Depression endogenous or psychotic	3. Hysteria	Hysterical*
		4. Obsessive compulsive disorder	Compulsive*
	c. Manic depressive psychosis	5. Depression reactive or neurotic	Alcohol/drug abuse
			Sexual deviance
	2. The schizophrenias	6. Others	Psychopathy
2. Chronic (largely irreversible) Dementia	a. Simple		
	b. Hebephrenic		
Examples senile dementia	c. Catatonic		
atherosclerotic dementia	d. Paranoid		
	e. Others		
Huntington's chorea ⎫ pre-	3. Paranoid states (excluding paranoid schizophrenia)		
Alzheimer's disease ⎬ senile			
Pick's disease ⎭ dementia			
		Psychosomatic Disorders Physical conditions with psychological overlay	

*Considered by the author to be more of a personality 'type' and characterised by withdrawal, mood swings, showy shallowness, compulsive behaviour respectively; not covered in detail in this book.

cation. It will not be universally acceptable and, although containing little original thought, must ultimately be seen as the responsibility of the author.

Disadvantages of classification

There are admittedly dangers in calling someone a schizophrenic or saying that they suffer from senile dementia. Stigma is still attached to psychiatric labels and the two categories cited are good examples of diagnoses which may give rise to exaggerated pessimism in those delegated their care. Such attitudes can encourage a self-fulfilling prophecy, making the likelihood of a positive outcome, even more remote.

Nevertheless, while bearing in mind the necessity of an individual nursing approach based on the observed needs of the patient, there seems to be some merit in referring to the traditional diagnoses. Certainly learners will hear them used.

The following section will therefore describe, with considerable emphasis on the role of the nurse, some of the more commonly recognised psychiatric syndromes.

In deference to those holding different views, and because it is essential that all learners should be aware of the existence of alternative schools of thought, Chapter 20 will be devoted to less traditional approaches.

The patient who is anxious
The patient who is phobic
The patient with unexplained bodily symptoms
The patient who is obsessional
The nurse and the neurotic patient
Psychosomatic disorders

11

The neuroses

Jamie (35 years old) has taken to pacing the office floor for hours on end as he wrestles with his business problems. At home he ruminates about his receding hairline and loose bowel movements. In bed he becomes increasingly aware of his heart beating, keeps his wife awake and finds sleep almost impossible. His marriage and performance at work are beginning to suffer.

Kathleen is terrified of cats.

Joan is 45 years old with a teenage family and an elderly mother. Recently following a bout of influenza she developed a weakness of the leg which has drastically curtailed her activities. A thorough medical examination has found no physical reason for this symptom.

Brian's fastidious lifestyle has gradually threatened to take over. Always meticulous regarding hygiene and office routine, he has now developed the habit of prolonged hand-washing following the handling of mail and must rise from his desk every few minutes to check his filing system.

Jamie, Kathleen, Joan and Brian do not suffer from psychiatric illness in the accepted sense of the word. They do not hear voices or see things which are not there. Many aspects of their daily living are unspectacular and their symptoms apart, they are remarkable only in their ordinariness. It is fashionable to describe such people as being *neurotic*.

Neuroses can be seen as immature attempts at adjusting to stress which tend to block or inhibit the individual's talents and instincts. Hallucinations or delusions are not present and the individual in many instances will appear essentially normal. The examples highlighted above, and shortly to be considered in greater detail, are in fact fairly extreme.

Few of us, if we are to be completely honest, could claim to be absolutely mature and well-adjusted. We may have an isolated fear or tendency to overreact to something others consider trivial, or perhaps we are merely overanxious to please our boss. At any rate, most of us have chinks in our psychological armour and could in certain circumstances be labelled neurotic. This does not mean that we are psychiatrically disturbed and most certainly does not imply that we require incarceration in a hospital.

Nevertheless, the ubiquitous nature of the neuroses has important implications for their management.

The nurse learner can expect to see comparatively few neurotic patients in hospital at any one time, even although some units do specialise in such treatment. Should an individual feel a need for medical help (and the majority will not) he will normally contact his family doctor. The GP depending on his interest and ability will himself deal with the bulk of his patients' psychological problems, which are said to make up a substantial part of his case load. Those who are referred to a psychiatrist are likely to be treated on an outpatient basis, with only the tip of the neurotic iceberg ever requiring hospitalisation.

It stands to reason that the minority who require to become inpatients tend to be the most seriously disabled and are therefore atypical.

Many people would argue that assigning a psychiatric label to what I have just described as being rather commonplace behaviour is unhelpful if not downright counterproductive.

Nevertheless, the following categories seem to occur sufficiently often to warrant a mention:

a. Patients may be anxious.
b. They may be phobic.
c. They may exhibit bodily symptoms in the absence of any apparent cause.
d. They may be obsessional.

PATIENTS WHO ARE ANXIOUS

Since all the above can be seen as attempts to ward off anxiety, (indeed the same has been said of mental illness in its entirety) the plight of these patients is perhaps more understandable than that of others.

A certain amount of anxiety is normal and perhaps even necessary.

We are anxious in case we do badly in examinations, so we study hard. The nurse learner may be anxious about her clinical assessments so applies herself diligently to the obvious benefit of her patients. Chip pans everywhere are gradually being thrown away as the nation belatedly becomes anxious about the amount of animal fats that is consumed.

Although closely aligned to *fear*, the two are not synonymous. Fear has an identifiable and realistic focus which is known to its victim. Fear amongst other things would prevent many of us from entering a bull ring or becoming involved in armed combat. If confronted by a desperado with a double barrelled shotgun, we would most certainly not be anxious — we would be terrified!

Anxiety, in fact, can be rather more vague, with the perceived threat being less obvious or physical in nature.

It may manifest itself for instance, before we make a speech, although the worst thing that could possibly happen would be to be laughed at or ignored. Nurses may be anxious when working with a clinical teacher, although the latter is now a domesticated species.

Being anxious also involves certain physical features that most of us can recognise. Palpitations, sweating of the palms, frequency of micturition, loose bowel movements and an inability to stay still are all commonly experienced by the anxious individual.

In its most extreme form anxiety can present as a *panic attack* in which the sufferer may experience dramatic physical symptoms and feelings of such terror that he is convinced he is about to die. Anxiety which is spread diffusely and does not focus on any single object or event, is said to be '*free floating*'.

> Jamie has always been over anxious. As a child he wet the bed until he was 11 years of age and suffered nightmares prior to examinations at school. Nevertheless, he gained good grades and joined a small firm of importers, with whom he has continued to be employed. He married at 30, his wife being of a similar age and they have a daughter, Beverley, aged 2½ years.
>
> Despite difficulty in disciplining staff and tremendous apprehension when called on to make major financial decisions, Jamie has found himself promoted to a position of some responsibility. Twice in the past — in his late teens and just prior to his marriage — he was treated with minor tranquillisers for an exacerbation of his chronic anxiety. At present he is coping less well than ever before.
>
> Jamie's GP has been unable to be of much assistance this time round and even the psychiatrist to whom he has been referred is beginning to see hospitalisation as inevitable.
>
> At the most basic level, hospitalisation would grant Jamie physical freedom from his business responsibilities and a much needed break from his marital tensions. His dosage of tranquillisers, could, with the additional supervision, be temporarily stepped up. It would be easier to ensure that he was eating and washing adequately and that any physical complaints be checked out by the doctor.

Absolutely vital as chemotherapy will initially be, Jamie and his wife are likely to need considerable psychological help once his initial overactivity and extreme anxiety begins to wane. Depending on the perceived problem, *psychotherapy*, (individual or group or *marital therapy*) may be suggested. Whatever the treatment, Jamie's intelligence and the support of his wife will give some cause for optimism, but his lifelong tendency towards anxiety will be hard to eradicate.

THE PATIENT WHO IS PHOBIC

We saw how Jamie could be described as displaying 'free floating' anxiety by reason of the fact that his feelings of apprehension were global.

Kathleen on the other hand, complains only of a fear of cats.

When anxiety, fear or apprehension is confined to only one, or a small number of situations, they are termed phobias. Kathleen's fear of cats and Mary's of aeroplanes are said to be *monosymptomatic*, that is only one thing is feared.

It is difficult to trace the cause of any particular phobia. Some people believe that it arises from an incident in the individual's past, when, perhaps in childhood, they may actually have been scratched by a cat, or frightened by a furry object. The incident although apparently forgotten may linger on in the unconscious.

On the other hand, phobias could be learned or copied from someone important to the sufferer. A young child who periodically witnesses her mother scream uncontrollably at the sight of a spider in the bath will grow up believing that this is a suitable response.

Analytically-orientated members of staff would postulate a more complex explanation. According to them the mental defence mechanism of *displacement* may be

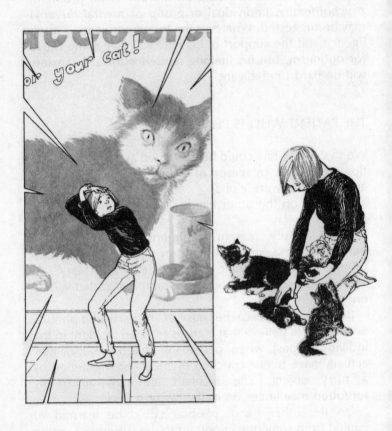

Agony . . .   and ecstasy.

involved, with the fear directed on the phobic object rightly belonging to something else, possibly less respectable. Thus a seemingly understandable fear of snakes, could they say, unconsciously represent a fear of the male sexual organ, or the sexual activity of mature adulthood.

Whatever the truth of the matter, the need for an explanation is doubtful. *Systematic desensitisation or flooding* (Ch. 7) enjoys considerable success in removing the symptoms while purposely ignoring the possible causes. It is now the treatment of choice for monosymptomatic phobias.

Unfortunately, monosymptomatic phobias in youthful, intelligent and well-motivated individuals are found mainly in the textbooks. In reality some complications are usually present. The patient may unwittingly be getting a degree of satisfaction from her symptoms, she may have a very dependent personality, or on closer observation, her anxiety may be much more widespread than at first thought.

Mrs T. attended hospital as a day patient. She complained only of a fear of shopping but seemed determined to overcome it. She appeared entirely suitable for treatment in a desensitisation programme which was immediately established. The nurse who had received guidance and encouragement from a part-time psychologist was to act as therapist. As each step in the hierarchy was attempted Mrs T. was asked to evaluate the amount of anxiety she felt by making a tick at the appropriate position on a 5 cm line.

Her initial response to treatment was quite spectacular. With virtually no setbacks she appeared to overcome her trepidations, reached the supermarket and brought back a sponge cake to celebrate!

Unfortunately Mrs T. lived in a town some distance away from the hospital and her new-found freedom from symptoms refused to be transferred to her usual shopping area. Sadly the whole procedure had to start again with the nurse this time travelling to Mrs T.'s home to supervise her treatment. Strangely, success now proved elusive with Mrs T. never reporting herself free of anxiety at any time. She failed to conquer the hierarchy and never reached the local supermarket unaccompanied.

Perhaps the nurse's observations of Mrs T.'s home circumstances helps explain matters. She lived with her husband, a fit man of 62 years of age, who had recently taken early retirement from his work. Their only daughter, married with two young children, lived nearby.

Mrs T.'s disability was entirely accepted by her family who went to considerable pains to organise their day around her needs. She was completely spared the hustle and bustle of everyday fetching and carrying and was very much the focus of everyone's attention. It seems that unconsciously at least, Mrs T. was unwilling to give up the perks of her condition, while her family too, colluded with her, possibly because of the gratification they received as carers.

The family dynamics although complicated, were well-established and 10 months later, Mrs T. showed only minimal improvement.

PATIENTS WHO EXHIBIT BODILY SYMPTOMS IN THE ABSENCE OF ANY APPARENT CAUSE.

Like Mrs T. such individuals may appear to get some benefit from their condition although they seem unaware of it. Historically they are an important group, since much of Freud's early work was carried out almost exclusively on females with unexplained physical symptoms.

This condition is known as *conversion* (psychological conflicts being converted into a physical complaint) but may be bracketed with dissociation (see below) and labelled *hysteria*.

> Joan, a single parent, had been increasingly under pressure. Her children, Peter, (19 years old) and Margaret (16 years old) were unemployed and generally unsympathetic. Her mother, who had recently come to stay, was proving very difficult, requiring increasing help with even the most simple activities of daily living.
>
> Following a short but incapacitating bout of influenza, Joan suddenly developed an alarming paresis of her right leg which she consequently dragged behind her. Exhaustive tests have ruled out any neurological or stroke-like involvement and the present diagnosis is one of hysteria.

Joan's apparent lack of concern about a complaint which would terrify most of us is typical of her condition, and is known by the French term *la belle indifference*. This involves a certain amount of dissociation, the other component of hysteria.

Dissociation involves a splitting off of painful emotion while the ability to function apparently normally remains. Amnesia, or memory loss, is a good example. On occasions this may take the form of *a fugue* when loss of memory occurs, during which time a journey is made. Individuals may suddenly 'come round' to discover themselves in a strange town, with absolutely no idea as to how they got there. To the casual observer, behaviour during these fugues usually appears normal. Fugues may explain the occasional newspaper reports of strangers turning up at airports or railway stations completely unaware of their identity or whereabouts. Even more spectacular but much less common is the dual or multiple personality, whereby the one individual can have two or more personalities functioning at different times, each entirely unaware of the other's existence.

Hysteria can ape almost any physical condition with headaches, sexual dysfunction, seizures or writer's cramp being common examples. Even blindness, deafness or aphasia can occasionally be traced to this source and regrettably, once an individual uses hysteria to cope with stress, he is likely to fall back on it repeatedly during subsequent difficult patches.

A related and modern phenomenon is termed *compensation neurosis*. Following an accident or other incident for which an insurance claim has been lodged, claimants may show a particularly negative response to the treatment of their injuries. At the present time this can be exaggerated by the long wait most actions have before reaching court and the symptoms are so ingrained as to become almost a way of life. In such cases it is hard to determine whether or not a degree of conscious malingering is involved and, of course, the level of financial award is likely to depend on how 'genuine' the symptoms are considered to be.

Prior to developing conversion or dissociative symptoms, many subsequent sufferers will have been observed to have a *hysterical personality*. This manifests itself in theatrical type behaviour with a shallow attractiveness. Such individuals require to be the centre of attraction and will use attention seeking methods and superficial seductiveness to achieve these ends. It is regrettable that their showy behaviour does not endear them to everyone in their environment.

Staff involved in the treatment of hysterical patients should remember that their behaviour, however dramatic or apparently contrived, represents an attempt to ward off (possibly unrecognised) anxiety. Measures which can reduce the anxiety would make such tactics redundant and in the long run may be more successful than the mere removal of symptoms by behaviourist methods.

PATIENTS WHO ARE OBSESSIONAL

This is a vivid example of how neurotic symptoms can be

used (often unsuccessfully) in an attempt to ward off anxiety. Obsessions commonly occur along with compulsions, and the term *obsessive compulsive neurosis* is often used to describe what can be an extremely incapacitating response to stress. The fact that the terms obsession and compulsion are familiar to the lay man and that the patient remains tentatively in touch with reality, should never be allowed to minimise the seriousness of the symptoms.

Obsessions, in the psychiatric context, are fixed or recurring thoughts in the person's mind, which he fully recognises as being abnormal. These thoughts cannot be dispelled for any length of time and because of their absurdity, may be very distressing. Thus an obscene word or phrase may continuously impinge on the awareness of an individual who consciously abhors such talk. He may have the recurring thought that his hands are being contaminated, that he may harm someone else, or that he has left the front door open.

A compulsion is an irresistible urge to carry out a piece of behaviour, which again may be realised to be illogical or absurd. Peace of mind will be unattainable however until the act has been performed and sadly, often this has no sooner been done, than it requires to be repeated. When obsessions and compulsions occur together, as they often do, they may involve endless rituals of hand washing, counting of instruments which could be used in an attack on others, or simply getting up to check the door lock.

Brian had always been meticulous and orderly. He could be described as being 'conscientious to a fault', always punctual, if somewhat constrained by his slavery to a routine. These qualities were part and parcel of Brian's make-up and have been described as evidence of an *'obsessional personality'*. Such traits can be of great value and may be sought after by an employer, but sadly a significant number of those who portray them will gradually develop a full blown, obsessive, compulsive neurosis.

For Brian, this arose during a particularly harsh winter, at a time when colds were prevelant. He became aware of the indisputable fact that his mail, as it travelled throughout the country, would be in contact with innumerable micro-organisms and was convinced that it represented a potent source of infection.

The fact that his colleagues handled their mail 'normally' and did not succumb to strange diseases, was acknowledged by Brian at a conscious level, but he rapidly developed a routine to safeguard himself against contamination.

This involved time-consuming hand washing rituals every time he touched anything which had been in the post. At home his distress was exacerbated if the envelopes were allowed to touch the floor and although a basket behind the letter box usually prevented this, the fact that a letter might somehow slip past it, was a further source of tremendous worry.

Hand washing momentarily relieved Brian's anxiety, but typically he would shortly be ruminating again. Had he missed any of his fingers? Was the soap contaminated? Perhaps to be really safe he should wash his hands *five* times after each contamination. Brian's other long-standing obsessional compulsive qualities seem to have increased too and particularly, his filing cabinet must constantly be tidied and retidied. But of course, much of the contents of his files have travelled through the mail and so his hand washing must recommence.

Brian can no longer carry out the duties which were previously so important to him and reluctantly he has had to accept hospitalisation.

Obsessive compulsive neurosis can be very resistant to treatment and can make 'normal life' virtually imposs-ible. Psychotherapy, the staple diet of the neurotic, is not very successful and the contribution of drugs or behaviour therapy is less than significant.

Symptoms may increase in intensity during times of obvious stress and decrease a little when things are more relaxed. Manipulation of external factors can therefore be important in allowing the individual to cope. A less stressful job may be considered, or home circumstances may be bolstered up as a first aid measure.

The therapeutic challenge presented by obsessive compulsive neurosis is exemplified by the fact that intractable cases may be occasionally treated with *psychosurgery*, one of the few occasions that such a drastic measure is taken in modern psychiatry.

Before leaving the neuroses it is necessary to mention depression. One school of thought believes that a specific condition known as *reactive* or *neurotic depression* exists and that this is qualitatively different from the more severe, endogenous depression. Depression is covered more fully in Chapter 12 — 'The Affective Disorders'.

THE NURSE AND THE NEUROTIC PATIENT

Many nurse learners may be surprised to discover that they find neurotic patients among the most difficult they are ever asked to care for. Regrettably, the word 'neurotic' has permeated into everyday usage. The lay person may apply it indiscriminately and with various degrees of accuracy. One thing is certain, it is never meant as a compliment! The neurotic patient often gives the impression of being more in control than he really is and this, along with his occasional 'showy' presentation, is not calculated to gain the sympathy of the busy nurse.

The nurse may be vaguely aware of sharing some of this patient's 'hang ups' and may feel irrationally aggrieved that she seems to be getting far less sympathy. Perhaps *transference* is again raising its head, with the nurse experiencing an upsurge of the emotion she first felt towards a sibling or childhood rival whom she considered to be favoured.

Psychotic patients on the other hand, who hear voices or are incapable of carrying out some basic task of daily living, are obviously more disturbed. Their needs, too, are more obvious, and although they will not necessarily be grateful, they are at least sufficiently 'different' to allow the nurse to carry out her task with a degree of emotional detachment.

The nurse who is aware of feelings of resentment or lack of sympathy towards a patient should acknowledge the fact (at least to herself), and try to reason why. She can take some consolation from the fact that it is utterly impossible to like everyone. Furthermore, any nurse who claims never to have negative feelings towards a patient must either be perfect, which is unlikely, or totally lacking in insight, which is sad. In any case, the bland quality of care such a nurse is likely to produce would be uninspired and liable to be lacking in the essential ingredient of empathy.

The fact that so far only negative feelings have been considered requires to be rectified. Many patients are intelligent, interesting and attractive, while nurses being human, share with the rest of the species the capacity to experience strong, positive feelings.

They have even been known to *'fall in love'*. It is difficult to generalise categorically about the forming of relationships with ex-patients (no doubt someone would write telling us of a 'perfect' marriage in which the couple met this way), but one thing is patently clear — special relationships cannot be allowed to develop on the *ward*. They are anti-therapeutic, unprofessional and being conceived in the unusual circumstances of the patient's present vulnerability, ill-advised. Usually the patient, who has all day to fantasise, will place much greater emphasis on his relationship with a nurse than vice versa. The nurse has many other patients to consider, and of course, the so-called 'home to go to'.

Patients who have struggled, perhaps throughout their life to form meaningful relationships and who feel that they are getting on well with the nurse, may be devastated to discover that it must end when they leave hospital. With this constantly in mind the nurse should never hold out any hope to the patient that their relationship can be a permanent one, but rather, from the start, must emphasise that it is a learning experience. Discharge and the weaning from a meaningful relationship should be planned well in advance and can form a vital part of the treatment programme.

The nurse learner cannot and should not be expected to cope with her emotions on her own. If staff *sensitivity groups* take place, and the atmosphere is such as to allow frank discussion, she may learn much in conversation with her colleagues. Alternatively, she may have to seek out a member of the ward or tutorial staff for guidance and in either case, she can feel perfectly justified with the demands she is making on their time. The development of self-awareness is an important part of the nurse's experience in psychiatry and she should not shirk from the opportunity when it affords itself.

Because of the immense variety of symptoms displayed by the neurotic patients, their care plans will be very much a personal thing.

Drug therapy may be less important than with some other categories of patients, although *minor tranquillisers* are widely prescribed. There is now an increased awareness that these drugs should not be used for prolonged periods and the whole team should realise that they should be constantly reviewed once the acute symptoms have subsided.

The psychological approach to treatment will be most prevalent, with, according to the needs of the patient and the particular orientation of the therapeutic team, individual psychotherapy, group psychotherapy or behaviour therapy being predominant. The need for physical nursing care will usually be minimal.

When *individual psychotherapy* is used, the nurse may feel excluded and must be prepared to be allocated an inferior position in the eyes of her patient. Alternatively, during a tricky phase of treatment, the patient may become very 'anti' her therapist and may try either to confide in the nurse or to glean from her any opinion or evidence which would cast doubts on his competence. The nurse has to avoid falling into this trap or becoming a buffer between therapist and patient. This is easier when the ward atmosphere encourages free flowing communication, staff attitudes are consistent and 'intrigues' are actively discouraged.

Most individual psychotherapy will be carried out on outpatients, who may or may not have had a previous spell in hospital, but who, in any case, will make no demands on the nurse.

PSYCHOSOMATIC DISORDERS

Long before she has reached her psychiatric module, the observant nurse will have noticed the importance of psychological factors in many of her patients' illnesses.

The term psychosomatic disorders describes a group of illnesses which, although demonstrably physical in nature, appears to be considerably influenced by the psychological state of the sufferer. Such conditions lie in the grey area between physical and psychiatric illness and depending on the interests and orientation of the examining doctor, greater or lesser recognition will be given to their psychological aspects. Some doctors would claim that almost any illness has a large psycho-logical overlay and may cite as evidence, the occasional dramatic improvement in inoperable cancer victims once their psychological needs have been catered for by hospice care.

Others of course hold the opposite view, believing that the mental state is relatively unimportant in all but cases of frank psychiatric illness. These days, this group is probably in the minority.

We have seen in Chapter 10 how some conditions such

as *bronchial asthma, duodenal ulcers* and certain *skin complaints* are widely accepted as having significant psychological involvement. Ulcerative colitis, a serious condition of the gastrointestinal tract involving disabling spells of passing bloody diarrhoea, is thought to be emotionally charged, as are some forms of dyspepsia or indigestion.

As a man, the author realises that he may be accused of all sorts of hideous sexual bias when venturing to talk of menstrual disorders. Nevertheless, *dysmenorrhoea* and the currently fasionable *premenstrual tension* (PMT) also often appear to be of psychosomatic origin. Myocardial infarction, the 'heart attack', which is a major killer in the UK seems to be particularly prevalent in ambitious, over-industrious types in 'stressful' occupations, although direct links are difficult to prove.

Psychosomatic disorders are not particularly common in psychiatric hospitals but will of course be seen from time to time. Rather, it is when she returns to her general wards that the nurse will come across these conditions and perhaps see them in a different light.

Anorexia nervosa is a disorder which is difficult to classify and which is often said to be psychosomatic. It is an extremely interesting condition which seems to be on the increase, occurring most often in girls of an age group similar to nurse learners. It is therefore considered worthy of a chapter of its own.

12

The affective disorders

The affective disorders is the term used in psychiatry to describe conditions characterised by an alteration in the *mood*. Affective disorders are important because they are relatively common and usually very treatable. In some ways they also seem understandable.

Examination failure, a broken romance or forced redundancy would make most people feel sad, while a pleasant meal, promotion at work or hitting the pools jackpot would do quite the opposite.

What is less understandable is the intensity of the emotion felt and on occasion the extent of the mood swings. Feeling low then can be perfectly normal, but to be totally crushed by a feeling of gloom and despondency from which there seems no escape, is not. Perhaps that's how it feels to be depressed.

Depression

Albert
Albert Brown was a 60 year-old security guard working in a large shopping precinct. He had lived alone

since the death of his wife from a brain tumour many years previously.

About 9 years ago, Albert was admitted to hospital with severe depression, but thankfully, in a matter of weeks, he responded to a course of ECT. He returned to work and seemed to progress satisfactorily. On two occasions since then, however, Albert has relapsed. 5 years ago he attended his GP for several months, having experienced an upsurge of his symptoms. Tricyclic antidepressant drugs and a great deal of support from his doctor pulled him through and once again, he returned to 'normal'.

Only last year he sought help yet again, spending 4 months in hospital, during at least part of which time he was said to be highly suicidal.

Today he is dead. Albert was found hanging from a rope tied to the handle and slung over the top of the door in the little flat where he lived. Hanging is final, Albert knew it to be so, and this time there could be no way back.

Mirabelle

Mirabelle has little in common with Albert. She lives in a comfortable part of suburbia with her husband and 11-year-old son. She is invited to lots of dinner parties, attends many coffee mornings and does occasional work for charity. Yet, Mirabelle, too, is depressed.

Her marriage has been less successful than it appears, her husband's business has unexpectedly floundered and she reacted with surprising intensity to the death of an aunt. She has come to believe that her lifestyle is shallow, her friends lacking in sincerity.

Following a family argument, Mirabelle swallowed some tablets washed down with strong lager. She was admitted briefly to the accident and emergency department, and now attends a psychiatrist weekly.

The similarity and differences between Albert and Mirabelle are important. Many people believe that there are two kinds of depression, *endogenous* and *reactive*. Albert would fit nicely into the endogenous bracket, while Mirabelle would be a good example of the reactive type.

However, it is said, perhaps ever more frequently, that

this divide is an arbitrary one and that any differences are in intensity rather than constitution. It is difficult to state categorically one way or another, but the nurse on the ward will be aware of a number of patients who seem to belong to one type or the other.

Albert's feeling of gloom and despondency would be of a level with which it is difficult to empathise and cheerful company would do little to improve matters. His whole bodily processes would be slowed up. He may be constipated, impotent (women may be amenorrhoeic) and slow in action and word. In fact his speech would be monosyllabic or he may be mute. These qualities hint at a physical cause and such a theory is given further credence by the often rapid response they make to the physical treatments of ECT or chemotherapy. The term endogenous means from within and is often used to imply that there is no obvious precipitating factor to explain the distress.

Delusions, often of a religious nature, or concerned with poverty or unworthiness, or involving the belief that the world is an extremely wicked place are common, leading to the alternative description of *psychotic* depression. Sleep disturbance is usually severe with early morning wakening. Sufferers may waken as early as 3 o'clock in the morning and be unable to fall asleep thereafter. Death by *suicide*, always a possibility, is most likely at this time.

Men more than women tend to suffer from this type of depression and a surprising number are of the so-called *pyknic body build*, with short, well-rounded trunk and short limbs.

Mirabelle, on the other hand, has no delusions and her sadness can be traced to obviously unpleasant features in her present environment. Hence, it can be termed neurotic or reactive depression. Sleep disturbance, if present, would present as difficulty in dropping off at night. Her mood may partially respond to cheerful companions or pleasant surroundings. This type of depression does not produce definite physical symptoms, although there may be complaints of vague aches or pains. Women rather than men tend to suffer from reactive depression.

Before leaving the question as to whether there is more than one type of depression, it is worth noting that the supposed differences can be even further clouded. Depression with the physical features of the so-called endogenous type may occasionally occur following an obvious precipitating event while the origins of some reactive type depressions may be obscure.

Involutional melancholia

This is a colourful expression, now seldom used, to describe a specific form of depression which first manifests itself in later middle age (the 'involutional' or menopausal period in women). Individuals, who until then had no relevant symptoms, develop a severe depression often accompanied by signs of agitation such as wringing the hands or pacing the floor. They are a severe suicidal risk. A feature of this condition is its usual dramatic response to ECT which is at its most effective in such cases.

Murder/suicide

From time to time a depressive illness will have the tragic end result of a parent (almost invariably the father) killing his family before committing suicide. The parent who may be very loving to his children becomes convinced that because of the unmitigated wickedness in the world, he is doing them all a favour.

In recent years, the press appears to have beome more sensitive to such tragedies and the banner headlines of a decade or two ago are now usually replaced by a brief statement that the bodies of, (for example) three children and a man have been found in a house, and that police enquiries have been completed. This low profile approach should be loudly applauded.

Hypomania

Most nurses may feel that it is appropriate to care for people with life-threatening depression — 'cheering them up' they may accept is part of their job. However, it may seem strange that people are admitted to hospital because of extreme happiness.

Full blown mania is less often seen nowadays because of treatment by chemotherapy but will be discussed later.

Hypomania, although less extreme, is nevertheless characterised by overactivity and increased rate of speech accompanied by a feeling of 'bonhomie' and extreme self-confidence. The happiness and mirth may be genuinely infectious.

Tony, a 39 year-old schoolteacher, was admitted to hospital as a compulsory patient only after a lengthy and by now familiar series of events had been allowed to unfold. In class, Tony is usually witty and entertaining, his pupils attentive. Gradually, his jokes began to take over his lectures, their content becoming ever more risqué, their delivery more rapid. His ability to concentrate wavered, his lessons became disjointed, until eventually they began to resemble a one man cabaret act. His colleagues, thrown slightly by his obvious feeling of well-being had their concerned attempts at intervention laughed off. Tony had never felt better!

Over the years, Tony's home life has become increasingly chaotic as he blunders from one financial crisis to the next. His wife and small daughter have recently left him, but remain very much a part of his intimate circle.

As his mood becomes ever more optimistic, so does his belief in his own business acumen. Just now it is computers.

Tony has invested in a battery of the most modern computer technology and talks grandiosely of setting up in business as a software programmer. Unfortunately, although he has already booked for a computer conference in Tel Aviv, next year, his plans have still to take off. He is hopelessly committed financially but lacks the concentration to do anything about it.

Hospitalisation often becomes necessary during hypomanic episodes to protect against financial disaster or public ridicule. This will usually be actively resisted or dismissed as outrageous by the victim, although it will be seen as absolutely essential by his family and friends.

MANIA

At any time, a patient who is suffering from hypomania may drift one stage further and develop full blown mania. His symptoms will become even more exaggerated, he will be completely unable to sit still, and will declaim loudly as if on a soap box. In days gone by, such patients sometimes died of exhaustion or because they had no time to eat, starvation.

Running closely parallel to the rate of activity will be the rate of speech, which will flit rapidly from subject to subject (flight of ideas) and on occasion will be entirely meaningless (word salad). A feature of the condition is a lack of inhibition coupled with complete frankness. The patient may throw off his clothes and/or make sexual offers or suggestions to whoever is in the vicinity. Cant will be immediately recognised and any insincerity will be spotted and loudly denounced.

Schoolboy jokes and puns may be repeatedly recited, while the mood swings from euphoria to ecstasy. Such delight will not be shared by his fellow patients, however, who are worthy of our deepest considerations.

MANIC DEPRESSIVE PSYCHOSIS

> Over the years, Jean has frequently been admitted to
> hospital. Her condition cannot be predicted but is usually
> dramatic in its severity. Now 53 years of age and with a keen
> interest in amateur dramatics, Jean has been known literally
> to swing from the curtains in sheer delight but has also
> come close to killing herself on at least three occasions.
>
> Yet for most of the time, Jean is quite well and holds down
> a fairly responsible job in the office of a firm of auctioneers.
> Recently, however, her breakdowns have been occurring
> more frequently and her periods of normal functioning have
> been shorter lasting.

Manic depressive psychosis is an affective disorder
characterised by mood swings of a degree not seen in
people who do not suffer from the condition. In
between acute episodes of mania or depression, the
mood can be stable and individuals can return to a
normal lifestyle with their intellectual reasoning unim-
paired. This is a mixed blessing, particularly after a
period of manic behaviour.

The nurse who may have had a little too much to drink
at a party can perhaps empathise with this plight. She may
be vaguely aware of having acted less discreetly than she
would have wished, or of having said things, that in the
cruel light of day, she realises would have been better
left unsaid. As next day she rather shamefacedly rejoins
her erstwhile fellow revellers, she, now sober, is unsure
of their reactions and worried lest she may have unwittingly caused offence.

Someone recovering from a manic episode (of much
longer duration than an evening of mild intoxication) will
experience similar trepidations but in a much more
exaggerated form. Since these individuals already seem
somehow to be predisposed towards depression, it is
hardly surprising that this may occur shortly after a
period of uninhibited mania.

Not all mood swings occur in rapid succession,

however. Some individuals can have 30 years between episodes by which time, the original one may even be forgotten.

An unfair irony seems to exist in that nobody appears to be able to enjoy the fleeting feelings of well-being associated with mania, without subsequently having to live through periods of depression, while the reverse, unfortunately often occurs. Many people suffer from recurrent depression without ever showing signs of mania. Sufferers from manic depressive psychosis prefer when their mood is slightly elevated but this is not shared by the relatives. They find the victim much easier to live with if he is slightly depressed.

The mood changes experienced by all of us can be seen as a normal reaction to the vagaries of daily living. Nevertheless, some of us may have amongst our acquaintances individuals whose mood swings seem more marked. Without missing work or requiring medical attention these people may commonly either be full of the joys or down in the dumps. They are said to have cyclothymic personalities, and although essentially 'normal', it seems reasonable to suggest that should they ever become acutely psychiatrically ill, they would most likely develop manic depressive psychosis.

The affective disorders — causative factors

The arguments about whether or not there are two kinds of depression, and the accuracy of the terms 'reactive' and 'endogenous' in some ways exemplifies the controversy of the affective disorders.

Manic depressive psychosis and the endogenous type of depression have a vague *hereditary* link. Offspring and siblings of sufferers are themselves significantly more likely to suffer, although the mode of inheritance is obscure. Consequently, it has not as yet been possible to identify with any degree of certainty the individuals most likely to succumb.

The response of some of the affective disorders to physical forms of treatment and the presence of definite bodily symptoms, suggests that a *physical* or *biochemical* factor may be involved. Indeed a diminished amount of brain amines has been identified in some cases, although why this should occur is uncertain.

Sometimes of course, depression can be seen purely as *an understandable reaction* to external events but, here again, caution is required. Other people living through apparently similar experiences seem able to shrug them off.

It appears that no single causative factor can be isolated. Individuals may be predisposed to affective disorders either by heredity or a particular form of brain metabolism but whether or not they develop full blown symptoms may depend on their life experiences and how in the past they learned to cope with stress. It seems futile to argue about the relative importance of each factor, which in any case, will differ from person to person.

Treatment

Depression is perhaps unique in the fact that the more severe the symptoms, the better the chance of recovery. The endogenous type, because of its aforementioned response to physical treatment has a good prognosis, (although it may well recur), but the reactive type may be longer lasting. Pills or electricity, after all, cannot make people like their husbands, or save them from bankruptcy.

In the affective disorders, ECT has an important role to play, especially in the type of depression known as involutional melancholia, where it can be a lifesaver.

Drugs, too, make a vital if less immediate intervention in depression and have revolutionised the care of the manic patient. Lithium salts as described elsewhere have an important preventative role in manic depression.

Depressions of apparently less severity, where environmental factors seem paramount, (reactive) do not respond so well to physical treatment. This is hardly surprising and perhaps psychotherapy offers most hope for this difficult therapeutic challenge.

The affective disorders and the nurse

Chapter 3 spotlights the role of the nurse in preventing suicide and in caring for the overactive patient. These are two of the most important symptoms of the affective disorders and the advice given there should be used as the basis for any care plan.

The maintenance of life, ensuring an adequate nutritional intake and preserving the dignity and individuality of the patient are of prime importance.

Less dramatically, the overall atmosphere of the ward can have an equally important role. The nurse must do her utmost to transmit her own quiet optimism while striving to ensure an environment for her patients, that is as non-threatening as possible. Enforced cheerfulness is unhelpful, although the reactive type depression may respond to pleasant surroundings. Often it is the nurse's ability merely to convey to the patient that he is valued and that his recovery is important to her that will make the greatest impression.

The nurse has one other vital role to play regarding the affective disorders — she must learn to spot them! Depression in particular can mimic a number of other conditions or may be largely asymptomatic. Since by definition, depression means misery and since we have seen that it can be so responsive to treatment, the nurse must ensure that it is recognised. Her unique relationship with her patients means she is in an ideal position to do just that.

13

The schizophrenias

Jennifer (22 years old), whom we met briefly in Chapter 2, has never worked. A quiet child, she had during adolescence gradually become ever more withdrawn, preferring to spend her time locked upstairs with her record player. Some years ago following the death of her father she had a brief spell in hospital but apart from that has survived at home. This has put a severe strain on her widowed mother who cannot understand Jennifer's apparent willingness to drift aimlessly with the tide and her lack of interest in 'normal' activities.

Although usually content to lounge about in bed, Jennifer who is physically very attractive, periodically takes to staying out at night. At these times she seems to enhance her limited income by sporadic prostitution.

John, on the other hand, appears to be almost an essential part of life in the large hospital that has been his home for 50 years. On admission as a 'certified' patient he had been convinced that his father was the Kaiser. He was kept in contact with a network of German spies who bombarded him with messages sent through the wind to his left shoulder blade.

His evil thoughts, John claimed, led to Hitler's invasion of Poland and subsequently the Second World War. During the war he remained in hospital but said he was working on 'top secret' missions for the Foreign Office. He was frequently observed, shouting in an agitated fashion towards the ceiling, from where on occasions, he seemed to get messages to which he listened intently.

Over the years John has changed considerably. He seldom talks of his strange ideas and works conscientiously, though over long, with the hospital porters. His unkempt appearance and shuffling gait tend to distinguish him from the members of staff to whom he is unquestionably subservient. His recent urinary incontinence does not seem to worry him although it could presumably jeopardise his continuing in the job he loves.

Jennifer and John are both said to be schizophrenic.

Schizophrenia is a complex, psychotic, condition which is poorly understood but which is a major contributor to severe psychiatric disorder. Approximately 0.85% of the population is said to suffer from schizophrenia and it is found in every known culture. Schizophrenia accounts for a large proportion of the long-term patients in any psychiatric hospital and constitutes one of medicine's greatest mysteries. It is responsible for a great deal of personal heartache and wasted potential.

Schizophrenic individuals are unfortunately considered by the lay public to have a 'split personality', but this does not mean that they conduct themselves in a Jekyll and Hyde manner. They tend to exhibit a definite blunting of emotions, with thought disorder and a general air of apathy. Although a clouding of consciousness and disorientation is normally absent, the personality shows definite signs of disintegration. It would therefore be preferable to speak of a fragmentation or splitting up *of* the personality.

Formerly known as *dementia praecox*, schizophrenia initially appears in young adults with the average age of onset being in the teens or early 20s. It seems probable that there is no single state of schizophrenia, but that rather there exists a group of related disorders which should more accurately be classified as '**the schizophrenias**'. Traditionally, four types of schizophrenia were described, and although this practice plays down the considerable overlap between categories and the difficulty in placing any individual correctly, the nurse learner will still hear them used. Consequently, it seems sensible to look in turn at simple, hebrephenic, catatonic and paranoid schizophrenia.

Simple schizophrenia

The onset of simple schizophrenia is usually insidious and at first symptoms may be mistaken for an exaggerated teenage 'phase'. A general lowering of all mental activity takes place with poverty of thought, action and affect. A gradual withdrawal into their own fantasy world is typical. Jennifer's case is typical of simple schizophrenia, in which hallucinations or delusions are seldom present.

Hospitalisation is not always required and is unlikely to be sought by the individual. Although the general aimlessness of their existence seems to call out for some sort of therapeutic intervention this is likely to be unsuccessful. Simple schizophrenics may lie in bed all day or alternatively may subsist in the shadowy periphery of normal life. Tramps, eccentrics, skid row alcoholics or petty criminals may on closer investigation show signs of simple schizophrenia. The outlook for recovery is usually unfavourable.

Hebephrenic schizophrenia

Gerry had been a textbook baby and a hard working, obedient child. However, as his secondary schooling proceeded he became more and more solitary, at first seeking refuge in his books, but later abandoning them completely. By the time he was 16, he had, at the expense of everything else, started on what he said was his life's work, a translation of the bible. He amassed a large number of religious and quasi-religious material in his bedroom and superficially seemed to be working hard. Closer examination, however, revealed that his activity was meaningless and he made no attempt to work constructively on his project.

Gerry arrived in hospital following a family upset, wearing a pair of sandals and an ill-fitting robe. Although dirty and dishevelled his likeness to some paintings of Jesus Christ was remarkable.

Gerry had fought with his father during an argument in which he claimed his father was one of the 'devil's co-operators'.

In hospital, he lay around giggling periodically in a fatuous and mirthless manner, freely announcing that he saw countless visions with whom he seemed to converse. He took no interest in the ward routine, frequently refused medication and seemed less and less able to carry out even the most basic activities of daily living.

After 14 months in hospital he has made little improvement and the future seems bleak.

Hebephrenic schizophrenia is characterised by an early, insidious onset and an inappropriate affect. Hallucinations are common and remissions seldom complete. A gradual deterioration is usually the rule, and therefore a large proportion of psychiatric long-term patients carry this diagnosis.

Catatonic schizophrenia

Marguerite, a final year social work student, had felt badly let down following the break up of a longstanding relationship with her boyfriend. In what may have been a deliberate effort to pick up the pieces she attended a wine bar with some friends who later planned to go on to a disco. During the early part of the evening Marguerite became separated from her companions and never in fact reached the disco.

On her way home some 3 hours later, one of her flatmates and a boyfriend saw Marguerite standing as if transfixed, staring at the pavement immediately outside the wine bar. Apparently she had stood there all evening oblivious of her surroundings and offering neither response nor explanation to the off duty policeman and his escort who were trying to be of some help.

On her subsequent admission to hospital, Marguerite was diagnosed as suffering from catatonic schizophrenia. She consistently refused to eat and made absolutely no attempt to care for herself in any way. She remained mute throughout the initial interview, unflinching even when approached with a pin, as if to be pricked.

After 3 months of intensive treatment, which included ECT Marguerite slowly began to improve. A period of bizarre conduct, which at one stage included the mimicking of movements made by others (*echopraxia*), followed, but gradually disappeared as she became more animated and alert.

She has been out of hospital for 6 months, is back sharing her flat and hopes to resume her studies in the near future.

Catatonic schizophrenia is perhaps seen less often nowadays. In its extreme form, catatonic stupor such as Marguerite's would alternate dramatically with periods of wild excitement. During these phases the patient's lack of insight and emotional inaccessability could make her extremely dangerous.

Despite its comparative rarity, it is likely that several patients in the long-term wards of a hospital may exhibit some signs of post catatonia. *Echopraxia*, as described above, may occur, as may *echolalia*, (the automatic repetition of words or phrases uttered in their presence). The ability of some patients to maintain their limbs in apparently uncomfortable or bizzare positions for a prolonged period is typical, and is termed *waxy flexibility*.

Catatonic schizophrenia, when compared with the other types, is more likely to arise as a result of a traumatic precipitating factor, with the onset being acute. These are favourable prognostic signs and the possibility of recovery from any single episode may be quite good. Relapses, however, are liable to occur.

Paranoid schizophrenia

Joe (39 years old) described himself as a nuclear physicist and mathematician, but stood in court accused of throwing petrol over the local police station in an attempt to set it alight. The petrol had been stolen from the adjacent garage where Joe worked as a part-time attendant at the pumps.

The local police, he said, were Chinese imposters who had secretly replaced the original force some time before. By using the electronic dial on his petrol pumps, these masqueraders could tune into his brain and extract secrets which would help them build a nuclear bomb.

Joe is unrepentant. 'Wrongs must be righted, and we must protect our weak ones,' he reasons. He angrily denies that there is anything wrong with him and resents the compulsory treatment ordered by the court. He blames it all on the Chinese, some of whom he claims have now infiltrated the hospital, 'to get even with him'. Because of the interest he feels the imposters are showering on him he is convinced he must be of extreme importance. He treats other patients and staff with the contemptuous disdain he believes their lowly status deserves.

He spends a great deal of his time in solitude scribbling furiously on mountains of paper which he covers with impressive looking mathematical symbols and equations. Although he insists this work is of grave national importance and far too complicated for all but the best brains to decipher, staff with a mathematical flair have established that it is entirely meaningless.

Despite his claims that he is being falsely imprisoned, he has made no attempt to escape and the greatest fear is that he may seek to retaliate against someone, staff or patient, in his immediate environment, who has become implicated in his elaborate delusional network.

Paranoid schizophrenia tends to appear in a slightly older age group, after the personality has had an opportunity to mature. Perhaps for this reason, people with the condition tend to present with more integrated personalities, appearing less bizarre or odd to the casual observer.

The main feature is their delusional system which can at times be very complex indeed. Individuals may believe that events portrayed on television or in the newspapers have a deep and personal significance for them (*ideas of reference*), or that they are being controlled by outside forces (*feelings of passivity*).

Thus an elderly lady on pass from hospital visited a horse trials and heard the commentator, on describing two horses, announce, 'This is a beautiful pair'. She believed he was announcing her engagement to a member of the aristocracy some 40 years her junior, and hurried to his country house to finalise the wedding plans!

Conversely, some people believe they have great power over external events and may hold themselves responsible for airline disasters or famines. When the UK changed to the decimal currency system in the early 1970s some long-term patients had difficulty in adjusting. At a ward meeting, one paranoid schizophrenic announced, 'I'm sorry, its all my fault. I told Harold (Wilson, former Prime Minister), that it would be a good idea. I was only joking, but he told the Queen!'

Claims to be familiar with well-known celebrities are common, and the use of the first name was no doubt meant to signify intimacy.

Because of their more intact personality, paranoid schizophrenics tend to deteriorate less dramatically than others and are therefore said to have a better prognosis. Nevertheless their delusions are usually fairly intransigent and complete reversal of symptoms is unlikely.

Other examples of the schizophrenias

Over and above the four traditional types of schizophrenia, the nurse learner is liable to come across a varied permutation of symptomatology and diagnostic labels. Some will be so atypical as to defy classification.

A *schizo-affective disorder*, however, is said to exisit when a patient who shows clear cut signs and symptoms of schizophrenia, is also subject to cyclical mood changes more appropriate to manic depressive psychosis (Ch. 12).

John (p. 198), whose acute symptoms are largely a

thing of the past, is correctly termed a chronic schizo-phrenic. However the unflattering description of *'burnt out'* schizophrenic is often used in such circumstances. Although colloquial and negative sounding, it vividly describes the state of flattened personality and lack of initiative which occurs in the absence of any florid symptomatology.

The schizophrenias — some possible causes

When the nurse considers the wide range of malfunc-tioning that can be encompassed in the label schizo-phrenia (not to mention the fact that it is probably several conditions anyway) she will not be surprised to learn that no single, clear-cut cause can be isolated. The following, however, may be significant.

Heredity

A definite hereditary factor exists, although the particular mode of inheritance and its overall importance is obscure. Individuals, whose family contains a schizo-phrenic, are much more likely to develop the condition themselves. This applies particularly to twins of those affected, even although they have been brought up separately from birth. This factor strongly suggests a hereditary rather than environmental explanation.

However, unlike haemophilia or Huntington's chorea, two distressing genetic disorders which follow a distinct pattern and where the chances of any unborn member of the family being a sufferer can be accurately forecast, schizophrenia is altogether less clear cut. It may be merely a predisposition to develop the condition if other, perhaps environmental, factors are also present that is inherited.

In any case the hereditary aspects seem important, should be noted, and deserve to be the subject of much further investigation.

Biological causes

Some people are convinced that the brain of schizophrenics must be different from that of the population at large. As diagnostic equipment becomes more precise and researchers more capable, they reason, these differences will be discovered and the mystery of schizophrenia unravelled. In the meantime, however, schizophrenic and non-schizophrenic brains seem remarkably similar.

One theory suggests that under stress, the schizophrenic brain may produce an abnormal, central transmitting substance and much research is currently channelled towards the investigation of this and other *biochemical* possibilities.

It has frequently been observed that an unusually high number of schizophrenics is of the so-called asthenic body build, that is, they are tall, angular and thin. This seems tantalising evidence of something, but as yet we know not what. Incidentally, those people tend to have a rather poor prognosis.

Environmental causes

These seem important. It is regrettable that many people seem to believe that only an environmental *or* a hereditary cause can be responsible. The opposite could be entirely true. It seems perfectly feasible that someone who is genetically predisposed to a condition could break down if subjected to adverse environmental factors, while others with no such tendency might remain well. When an obvious, traumatic event precipitates a sudden schizophrenic type response the prognosis may be marginally more optimistic.

A large percentage of schizophrenics are found living in low quality housing in and around the poorer parts of our inner cities. While many of us might have great difficulty in coping maturely with such an environment, it is too trite to say that the adverse living conditions are the cause of the schizophrenia.

A considerable number of schizophrenics drift towards these surroundings, perhaps in a search for anonymity, or maybe because they will find that others already there, are largely uncritical.

The family

The family is an important part of practically everyone's environment during their critical developmental stages. Consequently, it has been implicated in some causative theories. One theory has described the mothers of schizophrenics as having a greater than average propensity towards being cold, unfeeling individuals with a certain flair for distorting reality. This observation has led to the suggestion that certain mothers may be especially liable to produce schizophrenic children and to the coining of the phrase, schizophrenogenic mother. However, no scientific evidence is available to substantiate this theory and it has never been possible to identify such people in advance.

Consequently it has been largely discredited.

Some families are said to communicate in a very ambiguous manner. The child may constantly find himself the recipient of conflicting messages from each of his parents and is therefore likely to be in the wrong whichever way he turns. The withdrawal inherent in their schizophrenia can be seen as a psychological 'opting out' of an impossible situation.

A 'normal' response?

The theory that what we recognise as schizophrenia is actually a normal response to abnormal circumstances, has been expounded by some psychiatrists who would seek to deny the very existence of 'schizophrenic illness'. This cannot be dismissed out of hand. It is perhaps possible for us to imagine ourselves incarcerated in an unfriendly institution, unable to get out and surrounded by unpredictable companions. In such circumstances complete withdrawal from our surroundings might just make life bearable. But then of course, withdrawal is often used as evidence of schizophrenia.

Some of the more radical theories, both of schizophrenia and of psychiatric illness in its entirety, are presented briefly in Chapter 20.

Treatment of the schizophrenias

The treatment of the schizophrenias closely mirrors that of psychiatric disorders in their wider setting. Thus in the past it has included imprisonment, restraint, ridicule, surgery, ECT and drugs. Supportive psychotherapy and the initiative fostering approach of the therapeutic community have enjoyed some popularity as the philosophy of care has moved firmly in the direction of the prevention of chronicity and re-establishment in the community.

Several decades ago youngsters diagnosed as schizophrenic were hustled into hospital for what was in many instances, a virtual life sentence. In contrast, nowadays, the principle is largely one of hospitalisation for the acute episode only, followed by an early transfer to the community. In this way, individuals are given a greater responsibility for their own progress and former friends or neighbours are not allowed to dismiss them to a far corner of their memory.

The merit of today's approach can be assessed only after the passage of a suitable length of time. Hopefully as the more pathetic and deteriorated individuals in our long stay wards die, they will not be replaced by carbon copies. Instead perhaps, the future generations of elderly schizophrenics will be better integrated, show more initiative and be considerably less 'burnt out'.

The schizophrenias and the nurse

It is unhelpful for the nurse to refer to a patient as being schizophrenic and merely to plan his care accordingly. We can readily understand that someone who develops, for example, measles retains much of his individuality despite his diagnosis, and we are unlikely to be tempted simply to dismiss him as 'measlic' for the rest of his life. Surely the term schizophrenic is equally neglectful of the healthy properties which may flourish in our patients.

Chapter 3 explains how nurses should handle certain recurring situations, and it seems likely that many of the patients discussed there may have been labelled schizophrenic. This is important, but of course the first priority when dealing with, for instance, an agitated patient, is to help him relax, irrespective of what his main diagnosis may be.

Perhaps we can say that schizophrenic patients require empathic care but may shy away from too close a relationship. The young nurse who endeavours to be be friendly and warm to a patient in her care, may be startled at his rejection, but anything resembling intimacy may be too threatening for such a person. Many nurses have been aware of an apparent pane of glass between them and their patient, with whom meaningful rapport may be almost impossible. The intensity of the nurse/patient relationship may largely be controlled by the latter, and while the nurse learner does not have time on her side, she can, by maintaining a rather lower profile, encourage a more relaxed atmosphere.

Delusions and hallucinations feature prominently in many schizophrenic patients' repetoire. Such experiences are very real to the patient, and to deny their existence is seldom helpful. On the other hand there is little to be gained by actively encouraging comments on these breaks with reality, and it is pointless arguing about them. Neither the nurse nor the patient is likely to change their opinion. The only honest approach is to agree that what he is experiencing is very real, for the patient, but not to the nurse. Some schizophrenic patients may be petrified at the prospect of having their vaguely formed interpretations confirmed. For them, it may come as a great relief to have reality checked out and reinforced by the dissenting nurse.

14

Psychogeriatrics

THE DEMENTIAS

Mrs Barnes is usually charming and polite. In her 80s, she likes to sit on the seat at the window. She smiles when talking of Miss Buglass, her schoolteacher who 'ran off with a communist', but becomes silent if reminded of her son who died in the desert campaign.

She talks of shillings and half crowns and believes that she is in the local Conservative club. She dismisses with a trace of anger any suggestion that she may be in hospital.

Mrs Barnes suffers from a urinary complaint which means she has little warning before she must empty her bladder. More recently this has meant an increasing incidence of incontinence, which she usually denies. She seems to prefer sitting wet to allowing the nurse to provide her with a change of underclothes. At approximately 4 o'clock in the afternoon she invariably becomes agitated, insisting that she goes home to her mother whom she assures us will be anxiously awaiting her.

Mrs Barnes suffers from **senile dementia**, one of the more common psychiatric conditions affecting the elderly. Senile dementia arises as a result of an acceleration in the rate of the death of brain cells, for reasons which are not fully understood. Symptoms of senile dementia include memory impairment (especially for recent events), intellectual deterioration and disorientation for time, person and place. Emotional and social responses may or may not seem appropriate and as time passes, incontinence may develop. This condition is more commonly seen in women.

Atherosclerotic dementia which in appearance may be indistinguishable from senile dementia results from a gradual throttling of the brain by atheroma, a porridge-like substance. This adheres to the walls of the ageing arteries, reducing the lumen and subsequently decreasing the amount of oxygenated blood available to the vital neurones. This condition is more common in men and the onset may be gradual with periods of apparent remission.

PSEUDO DEMENTIA

Thankfully not all psychiatric disorders of the elderly are irreversible. Many conditions which may resemble dementia when first encountered may, when properly diagnosed, show a heartening response to treatment.

> Arthur arrived on the ward in an extremely unkempt condition. His clothes were literally falling apart and the accompanying smell suggested he was doubly incontinent. Nursing or medical histories were virtually impossible to obtain, his answers being slow, disjointed and seldom to the point. We established that he lived alone and he gave as his occupation, 'hunting rabbits'. He said he was 43 years old and was born in 1897.
>
> The police, who had been involved in Arthur's admission, confirmed that he lived in a dilapidated hovel in the countryside. Apart from dozens of empty soup cans, there were no signs of food, while even basic sanitary requirements seemed non-existent.
>
> Arthur scored very poorly on a mental functioning test, suggesting that his intellectual capacity had deteriorated to a marked extent. From a nursing point of view, most of the

activities of daily living were initially beyond him. He required a great deal of basic care.

Happily he was found to be suffering from *depression*. Depression is fairly common in the elderly and as in other age groups, usually responds well to treatment. And Arthur was certainly transformed. Good nursing care was responsible for feeding him up, controlling his incontinence, caring for his minor aches and pains and encouraging an interest in his surroundings. However, the contribution of the tricyclic, anti-depressant drugs which he was prescribed was probably crucial.

He appears to be of dull average intelligence and unsophisticated in the ways of the world. This will not change after 80 odd years but undoubtedly the misery to which he was subjected, has been largely eradicated.

It is difficult to know where Arthur goes from here. 'Home' seems entirely unsuitable but alternative accommodation is hard to come by. His wishes and background must also be kept in mind, and perhaps sheltered housing may eventually prove to be the answer. Certainly, a psychogeriatric ward is no longer appropriate.

Depression is only one condition which can closely resemble dementia in the elderly.

Paranoid disorders

Other disorders apart from paranoid schizophrenia, although not confined to the over 65s, commonly first appear as the individual gets older. These may be superimposed on what was always a rather suspicious personality and sometimes it can be extremely hard to decide when the stage of definite abnormality has been reached. This can be even more difficult when, as is often the case, the paranoid idea is encapsulated around one individual or set of circumstances.

Mrs Elliot was an exceptionally fit 93-year-old who was still largely able to cope on her own. Her memory and intellectual functioning had deteriorated mildly over a number of years but her only complaint was against her neighbours. Mrs Elliot protested appropriately and politely at the police station about the couple who inhabited the house next door. In particular, she objected to the fact that they held frequent all night parties where heavy drinking, sexual promiscuity and the smoking of cannabis commonly took place.

Anyone speaking to Mrs Elliot would have been convinced of her sincerity and sorry for her plight. Yet reality turned out to be very different. Mrs Elliot's neighbours, it transpired, were a mild mannered couple, themselves in their 70s, who regularly retired to bed immediately following the 'News at Ten'.

As we got to know her better, Mrs Elliot gradually discussed her life history with us. It was interesting to discover that, even in her young days she had always considered herself unlucky with neighbours, moving house on a number of occasions in an effort to rectify things.

On occasions, paranoid ideas may sound so credible as to be extremely difficult either to prove or disprove while at other times they may be very fanciful indeed. Old people may believe neighbours are trying to gas them through the floor boards, or have wired up their beds to the electricity mains and may complain loud and often to the police. Regrettably if they consider that the police are taking no action they may be tempted to take the law into their own hands.

Paranoid symptoms in the eldery are notoriously difficult to treat, although some individuals, realising that they are not being believed, will learn to keep their ideas to themselves. Careful probing by the psychiatrist, however, would reveal that they are lurking, undiminished just below the surface. Sometimes old people living alone suffer *sensory deprivation*, with little going on around them to occupy their mind. Admission to the more sociable surroundings of a hospital, where there is plenty activity, may prove stimulating and the need for distorting reality may disappear.

The careful assessment of all old people admitted to hospital must be a priority. Capitalist society tends not to respect the elderly as they have ceased to be productive, thus they are more likely than others to be written off as incurable. Symptoms of normal ageing such as a degree of inflexibility or some short-term forgetfulness can be overemphasised and presented as a psychiatric disorder. This is inaccurate and unhelpful.

NON-NURSING CARE OF THE ELDERLY PSYCHIATRICALLY DISORDERED

This includes the making of accurate diagnosis and treating remedial conditions. In addition supporting therapies, much as for other older people, require to be provided, as does the maintaining of appropriately positive attitudes.

Diagnosis and treatment

Depression is the prime example, but other conditions such as trauma, thyroid problems or chest infections can also easily be overlooked. Medical staff have in their repetoire suitable treatments for such conditions and the results may be gratifying. Aggressive medical treatment has so far proved inconclusive in dementia and although vasodilators should in theory help increase the supply of oxygenated blood to the brain cells, results to date have been disappointing.

Multiple pathology

Is a well-recognised accompaniment of old age, and commonly the old person may suffer from a variety of aches and pains throughout their body. These must be actively sought out and when possible treated, irrespective of the individual's age or mental state.

Support therapies

These include physiotherapy, chiropody and lunch clubs, which, although not directly combating dementia are of proven value to old people in more favourable circumstances. If available, they should be prescribed when the need arises. Occupational therapists may be actively involved in assessment, reality orientation or reminiscence sessions, while some social workers will have special interest or training in psychogeriatrics.

Attitudes

The term 'the elderly', although widely used, is without qualification, not a helpful one. If, as is so often the case, it is applied to everyone between 65 and 95 years of age it becomes meaningless since the difference in individuals in such a cohort would be absolutely tremendous. The Americans have coined the term *ageism* to describe the prejudices and mythologies to which we subject our elders. Although less widely recognised this may be as potent a force as racism or sexism and leads to the passing of the years being automatically equated with physical and mental infirmity and asexuality. This can lead to undue pessimism in our dealings with old people, who if eccentric, may be classed as being slightly deranged, or if mildly demented, being branded as beyond hope.

Professionals, whatever their speciality, are ideally placed to dispel within their own circle, these damaging stereotypes.

THE NURSE AND THE PSYCHOGERIATRIC PATIENT

The number of over 75 year olds in the UK is expected to rise until well into the next century, so we can safely assume that the demand for psychogeriatric nursing care will also increase. This means that nurses trained and working in psychiatry, can sooner or later, expect to spend some time in this speciality.

The psychogeriatric patient requires physical nursing care of at least as high a standard as anyone else. Of this there can be no argument. Sadly, on what is hopefully the rare occasions that nurses fail to provide adequate care, the elderly mentally infirm, along with the mentally handicapped, seem most likely to suffer.

'Sans Everything' a factual account of the experience of an old person in hospital, rocked the nursing world in the late 1960s, highlighting many deficiencies in care and patient abuse in one hospital at that time. Perhaps the most spine-chilling feature of the book was the fact that the inadequacies reported could so easily be repeated elsewhere. It remains essential reading for everyone involved in caring for the elderly mentally infirm.

In their attempt to achieve competence in the activities of daily living psychogeriatric patients may be uniquely disadvantaged. The ravages of *multiple pathology* described above, means they are liable to require assistance with the most basic of tasks such as eating and keeping warm. In addition, their superimposed and usually irreversible, psychiatric disorder, will greatly complicate matters.

Nurses training for the general register will have already nursed old people either in a special module or in medical or surgical wards. In this a textbook on psychiatric nursing it is not our plan to reiterate what has been taught elsewhere, rather we shall merely draw attention to its relevance.

Areas more specific to the old person with psychiatric disorders will be dealt with below.

Maintaining a safe and pleasant environment

Until recently psychogeriatric patients were commonly nursed in 19th century buildings. These were usually part of the old asylums, or in establishments originally built to cater for the unfortunates who fell foul of the poor law — the parish workhouse. In either case the buildings were gaunt and austere and had an unenviable reputation amongst the old people of the district. The stigma of dying in such places meant that hospitalisation was resisted until the very last minute, usually long after any hope of arresting the deterioration had vanished.

Many people can testify that efficient and kindly care did take place in such architectural relics, but undoubtedly such an environment was far from ideal. Privacy was hard to achieve, bathing and toilet facilities were usually inadequate, while the large and often overcrowded wards encouraged, what in modern parlance, is usually called *task-orientated care*.

Perhaps the provision of single storey, custom-built units with bright and compact day areas and full supporting services, seems a panacea. Certainly many such establishments have mushroomed over the past 20 years before economic reality and cutbacks began to bite.

Modern improvements include the installation of lifts, doors wide enough to accommodate wheelchairs, roomy bathrooms, small bays or cubicles and double glazing. Particularly fortunate establishments have facilities for hairdressing, chiropody, physiotherapy and occupational therapy contained on the premises with experienced staff around to take advantage of them.

Yet architectural splendour is only half the battle. Repeatedly it is found that the best nursing care does not necessarily take place in the most modern buildings. The enthusiasm and innovation of a truly interested nurse is the patient's best bet. Such nurses can do much to make up for the shortcomings of their surroundings and prove that nursing excellence can occur where conditions are far from ideal.

Safety

Those responsible for the elderly who suffer from psychiatric disorders must make a major policy decision.

Should their charges be confined to the relative safety of geriatric chairs with perhaps the added precaution of medically approved sedation, or should they be encouraged to remain as mobile as possible for as long as possible? Overt physical restraint is banned, but a combination of drugs and the rather dubious table fastenings on some chairs can make it very difficult for their incumbents to get about. The risk of injury is reduced, but is the price too high?

The alternative is to allow relatively unrestricted but carefully supervised movement throughout the ward. The attendant risks are obviously very much greater but the psychological and physical benefits to the majority may mean that they are justified. The answer may lie somewhere in-between. Preventable accidents should never be explained away or written off as just one of those things, but equally, the mere possibility that they may occur should not be used as an excuse for immobilising wandering patients.

Basic safety measures applicable to all wards take on a new significance when the patients are both frail and psychiatrically impaired. For a combination of reasons these patients will be less able to spot potential hazards in their path, so possible obstacles like walking aids, electric flexes or frayed carpets must not be allowed to go unchecked.

Fires and radiators must be carefully guarded, especially as some patients may have very little sensation in some parts of their limbs and may seriously injure themselves without realising it. Bleaches and cleaning fluids must be locked away and the kitchen containing such risk factors as cookers and boiling water should be out of bounds. Beds, if adjustable, should be turned *low*, therefore reducing the risk of injury should the occupant be unfortunate enough to fall out.

The orientating effect of conspicuous *sign posting* has been discussed in Chapter 3 and, by reducing the amount of aimless wandering, such measures must positively influence the accident rate.

Some patients are unfortunately always on the go. They are the people who will refuse to sit down and on whom, even drugs have little effect. In the absence of any trite answers it is worth emphasising the need to take a careful nursing history in such cases. Is there an explanation, or even a solution? Sometimes there is not, but a programme of behaviour therapy usually under the direction of a clinical psychologist can sometimes reduce the amount of activity, or as they may be tempted to describe it, 'undesirable behaviour'.

Social/recreational stimulation

The term stimulation is preferred to therapy here, as there is no reason why old people should be subjected to a gruelling circuit of activity merely in the name of fun. Yet recreation and social interaction is important on at least two counts.

1. It is stimulating. Even a fairly passive pursuit such as watching videos has definite orientation value if, for instance, it can be established that this takes place on Tuesdays and Fridays at 3 p.m. in the sitting room. Such highlights split the week up and provide nurses and patients with a mutual talking point. Instead of each day being a grey repetition of what went before, the nurse can now say to her forgetful patients, things like 'This is Thursday afternoon, Mr Black. This time tomorrow we will be watching *The Sound of Music.*' This will be effective for some patients, some of the time.

Other activities requiring more active participation may have additional benefits. *Bingo* exercises the ability to differentiate between numbers and emphasises the need to concentrate, while dancing or simple *calisthenics* (light exercises to music) introduces a degree of physical involvement.

2. It is enjoyable. We have established that many of the inhabitants of our psychogeriatric wards will be there for a long time. In that case they are morally entitled to as enjoyable a lifestyle as is possible and entertainment is perfectly justifiable in its own right, irrespective of any 'therapeutic' value it may have.

A word of caution is required. Recreation is a personal thing and difficult to organise in batches. Bingo for some will be a welcome reminder of past pleasures, while for others it will signify mass boredom. Basket-weaving, too, will find favour in certain quarters, but can also be seen by a reluctant participant as damning evidence of how far he has fallen.

As we have seen, most psychiatric hospitals employ *social/recreational therapists* and these are likely to be psychiatrically trained nurses. Their responsibilities will cover the whole of the hospital and they will co-ordinate activities for all age groups. The organisation of social and recreational programmes will be largely theirs, although they will have to work closely with nurses at ward level. The social/recreational therapist cannot work in a vacuum and every member of staff must be aware of the possibilities in this field. Their enthusastic involvement may greatly enrich their patients' quality of life.

DISPOSAL

We have tried throughout this chapter to dispel the image of psychogeriatrics as being hopeless, helpless individuals slowly stagnating in an unfortunate environment. Nurses familiar with general nursing could readily testify that elderly patients tend to remain in hospital longer, often claiming a bed in an acute area which could possibly be more profitably used by someone else. This problem applies equally to psychogeriatrics.

Ideally, patients should be admitted to a short-term *assessment ward* where a sufficient number of experienced staff will be available to offer, short-term care, acute treatment and a realistic assessment of the likely outcome.

The success of assessment wards or units depends largely on the amount of *back-up* facilities available elsewhere. Such facilities should include rehabilitation units, where the aim is to restore the old person to a significant degree of dependence, long-term wards and community facilities such as sheltered housing, hostels or old folk's homes.

Movement between these various establishments should be flexible and two-way. A resident in a long-term ward may surprise everyone and prove able to be transferred to sheltered housing, while someone in an old folk's home may deteriorate rapidly to the stage where she requires long-term care and attention. It is desirable that such transfers occur quickly and with the minimum of political manoeuvres since the patient's lifestyle, not the administrative convenience, is what matters. The situation where some old people are long-term patients in a psychogeriatric ward because 'they have nowhere to go' is a sickening reflection on the priorities of modern day society. It should not be tolerated.

Summary

The care of old people with psychiatric disorders is a nursing speciality. The number of such people is growing rapidly. Reversible conditions should be actively sought out and treated, but unfortunately many elderly psychiatric patients suffer from a degenerative condition — one of the dementias.

Working in this speciality has traditionally not been popular. In the past it has sometimes been said that nurses have been allocated work with the elderly as a means of punishment and whatever the truth in this, it is true that the apparently more able often sought employment elsewhere.

This, however, may change. As nurse training increasingly encompasses the care of the elderly and the mentally disordered it seems reasonable to assume that some nurses will discover their niche in psychogeriatrics. There is some indication of an upsurge in interest in post-basic courses in caring for the elderly. This in turn may stimulate interest in nurses already working in the area and boost their status in the eyes of the profession. Certainly their contribution is highly significant and much needed.

SUGGESTED READING

Pitt B 1982 Psychogeriatrics, 2nd edn. Churchill Livingstone, Edinburgh
Robb B 1967 Sans Everything, a case to answer. Nelson, London

Alcohol abuse
Drug abuse
Sexual deviancy
The psychopath
Treatments
Nursing the patient with a personality disorder

15

Personality disorders

Not all neurosis presents itself in a straightforward fashion as in a phobia or a hysterical paralysis. Many people, while displaying little in the way of definite symptomatology, still manage to conduct their lifestyle in such a chaotic manner as to differentiate them substantially from their fellow beings.

When their immature strivings to cope with life's stresses and strains are well established and infringe on a large chunk of their lifestyle they are said to have a *personality disorder*. The term character neurosis (as opposed to the symptom neuroses of Chapter 11) is analogous with personality disorder.

Ascribing personality disorders to individuals is obviously a very subjective exercise, as the perfect, or ideal personality almost certainly does not exist. Mild eccentrics or a variety of local 'characters' could be included but it seems sensible to confine the term to those whose personalities are either upsetting for themselves or disruptive to society.

Because personality traits are deeply ingrained and long standing, they are often not recognised by their owner as being unusual. Consequently, he may not see the need for 'treatment' and may even actively resist it.

In this chapter we will look at alcohol and drug abusers, sexual deviants and 'psychopaths'.

ALCOHOL ABUSE

Mr Rawlings is a successful accountant and a member of two exclusive golf clubs. Since leaving university 17 years ago he has driven himself hard in order to 'get on'. His outgoing personality means that ever since he was a junior member of the firm he has been involved in providing hospitality for valued clients.

2 years ago, following an emergency operation on a duodenal ulcer, Mr Rawlings became tremulous and agitated. He complained to the nurse about a filthy pillow slip which to her eyes seemed clean, and then he mistook the young doctor for a steward at the golf club. He was immediately treated with vitamins and tranquillisers and thankfully the incident proved merely a hiccup on his road to a successful recovery. On his discharge, it was advised that he cut down on his alcohol intake, but he was pronounced cured.

Mr Rawlings is nobody's idea of an alcoholic but yet undoubtedly, following his enforced abstinence in hospital, he came close to developing *delirium tremens* (the 'DTs' which are associated with tremulousness, agitation and visual hallucinations and may be a feature of sudden alcohol withdrawal).

His drinking usually starts about midday (although secretly he has had one on the occasional morning, 'to get me going'). It is customary for him to entertain clients over sometimes protracted expense account lunches. Normally he stops at his golf club for several drinks with his friends before going home for dinner with which he has wine. The rest of the evening is spent drinking in a civilised manner at a nearby hotel. He leaves just before midnight and walks home apparently sober.

Mr Rawlings is an alcoholic. Cushioned by an expense account and a good salary he has yet to face the full financial implications of his addiction, although his health has already been affected. Currently he is separated from his wife for reasons about which he is rather vague. He seems strangely non-plussed about this but more concerned about the fact that his promised partnership in the firm has not been forthcoming.

Mr Rawlings is typical of a large army of alcohol abusers who somehow seem to be getting away with it! He would strongly deny his addiction and therefore sees any suggestions that he seeks treatment as ludicrous. To him, alcoholics belong in the gutter and he has still some distance to go.

> Vince is almost there. A former steel worker in a now closed shipyard, his story seems much more typical.
>
> He started drinking with the lads shortly after leaving school, at first concentrating on the weekends prior to going dancing or to a football match. As the yard flourished, Vince spent more and more time and money in the nearby public houses, revelling in the uncritical camaraderie he found with his mates. After years of squabbling, culminating in months of failing to pay his board and lodgings he was thrown out by his widowed mother with whom he had always lived.
>
> There gradually followed a downward spiral of cheaper, less desirable lodgings, seedy public houses, and scruffier companions. He has been fined for urinating in a bus shelter, breach of the peace and more recently for being drunk and incapable.
>
> When the shipyard closed rendering him unemployed, he welcomed the longer drinking time it gave him. As his income became smaller, he spent more money on alcohol, electing eventually to economise by sleeping rough. Aged 43 years, he has had three spells in hospital as a result of alcoholism and one with bronchitis.

As examples of alcoholics, Mr Rawlings and Vince are at opposite extremes. Women, too, are affected and an ever increasing number of teenagers are showing signs of addiction.

Almost universally used to aid relaxation, to celebrate life's minor successes and as a symbol of our hospitality, alcohol nevertheless is a serious problem with which a sizeable number of individuals just cannot cope.

Why certain people become alcoholics is difficult to ascertain. It tends to run in families, but seems more likely to be copied or learned rather than inherited. No apparent biological factor has been demonstrated and the theory that alcoholics are somehow allergic to alcohol has been well and truly refuted. Some people drink as a symptom of another disorder, as for instance the schizophrenic who seeks solace from his voices.

Perhaps alcohol seems to offer an easy solution for individuals who are unable to face up to the rigours of everyday life. As a 'social anaesthetic', however, it is short-acting and dangerous. Alcoholics are prone to a variety of gastrointestinal disorders, vitamin deficiencies, peripheral neuritis, cirrhosis of the liver and psychological or social disintegration.

Korsakov's syndrome combines peripheral neuritis with gross memory impairment and a tendency to confabulate, that is, fill in the gaps with what seems to be suitable fabrications.

The problem affects all levels of society and it is unhelpful to consider alcoholism as purely the prerogative of the down and out. Those presenting for treatment in hospital represent merely the tip of the iceberg and a much greater number will be receiving no help whatsoever. Some may be seeing their GP or other agencies in the community.

The treatment of the alcoholic can ideally be described in two stages:

1. they must be withdrawn from alcohol (dried out) and physically patched up, and
2. while remaining abstinent, they should be helped to explore the reasons for their addiction and to try to restructure a daily routine which is not dominated by a need to acquire the next drink.

Traditionally, many alcoholics receive only the first stage of treatment, with the more intense second stage being reserved for those more promising cases with insight willpower and a genuine wish to change. Drugs such as disulfiram (Antabuse) or citrated calcium carbimide (Abstem) can help the alcoholic abstain since, if taken regularly, they produce unpleasant physical side-effects if alcohol is subsequently consumed within 24 hours.

Alcoholics Anonymous (AA)

AA was founded in America by Bill W. and Dr Bob and has proved invaluable to many alcoholics the world over. Based on the principle of self-help, members must accept that they are powerless over alcohol and must abstain completely. Many alcoholics find it much easier to relate to fellow alcoholics than to medical or nursing staff whom they may perceive as being critical or simply ill-informed. Some potential members can be put off by AA's quasi-religious style, but nevertheless it does excellent work and the nurse can feel safe in recommending it to her patients.

The nurse and the alcoholic

Nursing the alcoholic requires a rare mixture of empathy and firmness, an approach which is equally necessary for dealing with other patients described below. A detailed review of the nursing care will therefore be held over to the end of the chapter.

DRUG ABUSE

Jimmy 'mainlines' heroin and at 22 years of age is a physical disaster. He has a long criminal record and a short life expectancy. Peter, a 19-year-old dental student, smokes pot, to the chagrin of his mother who reaches for her Valium. Barry sniffs glue behind the bicycle sheds at school.

It is fashionable but nevertheless accurate to say that drug abuse has reached epidemic proportions in parts of the Western world. Less obvious is the wide range of individuals who can be classified under the umbrella of drug abuser and the diversity of the needs they exhibit. In an area where the ground rules change so rapidly it is impossible to give an overview that is completely up-to-date. The following therefore are purely examples.

'Hard' drugs such as the opiates and their derivatives which include morphine and heroin are, with some justification, the headline grabbers. Here physical dependency can occur very rapidly and death may result from a variety of complications. The use of unsterile and communal needles and syringes constitutes a major health hazard to these people. Although in the UK it is possible for an addict to register and thus legally receive a supply of his drugs, the scene is inextricably linked with the criminal world.

Young adults are particularly prone to become 'hooked' on hard drugs but it is very difficult to detect in advance those most at risk.

In hospital, the hard drug user is likely to seem totally immersed in his habit. Although plausible and capable of superficial charm, he will be devious and amoral. Denied his drug in sufficient quantities he will become agitated and desperate enough to do anything.

Nurses must take great care to lock away all syringes, used or otherwise, and should be on the constant lookout for drugs which may be secreted in a variety of ingenious hiding places. Addicts may attempt to leave the ward in order to get a 'fix' or may persuade their (possibly like-minded) visitors to smuggle drugs into the hospital.

It seems likely that this deterioration in personality and trustworthiness is a result, not of any physiological attributes of the drug, but of the deceit and criminal activities necessary to maintain a habit which requires a vast amount of money each day.

Less dramatic than the opiates are a variety of other substances which are prone to abuse. *Hallucinogens*, of which lysergic acid (LSD) is the best known, have a mind-altering effect which on occasions can mimic schizophrenia. First popular in the 1960s, it is said that the individual does not become addicted to LSD but he certainly becomes very preoccupied with its properties. Alarming features of LSD are the 'bad trip' when frightening and unpleasant sensations are experienced, and the 'flash back' phenomenon when users can suddenly re-experience the 'trip' without taking further supplies.

Amphetamines are taken in the mistaken belief that they increase concentration and give added vigour, when in fact they merely elevate the mood for a limited period. Prolonged use may result in a full blown psychosis in which paranoid features are prominent. Amphetamines are sometimes mixed with cocaine, a hard drug enjoying some popularity. Amphetamines have been used therapeutically as an aid to slimming because of their appetite-depressant effect, but their habit-forming properties make this undesirable. They seem most attractive to adolescent thrill seekers and obsese women.

Barbiturates medically prescribed were at one time a major source of drug dependence by groups of people far removed from the popular image of the 'junkie'. These were often middle-aged women, and although GPs have now voluntarily reduced the number of barbiturates they prescribe, their place has partially been taken by minor tranquillisers which, although physically safer in overdose, may still be habit forming. They are perhaps best prescribed to help cope with acute episodes of emotional dysfunction and their long-term use should be discouraged.

Cannabis or marijuana has achieved a degree of notoriety because of its widespread use and a well-orchestrated campaign for its legalisation. Cannabis is widely believed to be fairly innocuous and the main danger in its use may be the fact that it appeals to a young and impressionable section of the community who may be tempted to experiment with harder drugs as a result of initially smoking cannabis. Supporters of legalising cannabis point out that the law, as it stands, makes criminals of many potentially useful members of society. It forces them to mix in an environment where harder drugs are available and crime is rife. Those in favour of the status quo cite the damage to individuals brought about by tobacco and alcohol and see no merit in deliberately introducing another temptation for the weak willed.

Cannabis smokers are unlikely to present for treatment of their own free will and may only be seen by psychiatric nurses if they have become involved with the police.

Glue sniffing is a term used to describe the abuse of a whole range of solvents, sometimes by very young school children. Unfortunately the habit shows signs of being much more than a short-lived craze and a considerable number of deaths has occurred. Everyone connected with young people should be on the lookout for any hint that glue sniffing is taking place and any attempt at glamourising it should be rapidly put down.

The aforementioned description of drug abuse is complicated by the fact that individuals may frequently abuse more than one substance (including alcohol), depending on what is available and in fashion.

Treatment

This involves weaning the abuser from his habit and attempting to replace, with something else, his total preoccupation with drugs. Withdrawal from hard drugs will precipitate severe physical symptoms, and is best brought about by gradually substituting them for a less noxious alternative. With other types of drugs, the craving will be less severe, but anyone who has tried to give up cigarette smoking after the habit has become established will be aware of the magnitude of the task. The relapse rate, therefore, is notoriously high and the presence on the ward of a drug abuser may arouse great ambivalence in the staff.

General management problems which may affect the nurse is discussed at the end of the chapter.

SEXUAL DEVIANCY

This term has an almost old fashioned ring to it nowadays, as the wide diversity of sexual activity indulged in by some people is slowly realised. For instance, life is perhaps easier for the homosexual than at any time in the past. There seems to be a trend towards regarding anything practised between consenting adults in private as acceptable. However, some people's sexual inclinations and orientation are such that they will invariably find themselves in sharp conflict with society and the law.

Paedophiles, who desire sexual relationships with children, are universally abhorred (but must be accepted and cared for by the nurse) while *exhibitionists* — men who feel compelled to show their penis to women, but who normally refrain from any closer contact — are prosecuted with a vigour out of all proportion to their rather pathetic offence.

A tragic feature of many so-called deviancies is their apparently compulsive nature. Readers of a certain type of newspaper will be very familiar with tales of respectable businessmen or public figures, well able to calculate the effect of their action, losing their position, family and integrity as a result of momentarily giving in to their unacceptable desires.

Unlike many personality disordered individuals, sexual offenders usually retain the capacity to experience guilt. Consequently they may suffer unrelenting torment and shame from their own conscience as well as from external sources.

Some sexual offenders may benefit from a course of aversion or behaviour therapy but many eventually relapse.

THE PSYCHOPATH

The psychopath, or as he is frequently called: the socio-path, is one of life's enigmas. Charming but heartless, superficially attractive but cold, sane but capable of acts which can only be described as madness.

The Mental Health Act, England and Wales, 1983, revised the definition of the psychopath as follows: 'persistent disorders of mind (whether or not including significant impairment of intelligence) which result in abnormally aggressive or seriously irresponsible conduct on the part of the patient.'

The McCords state: 'The psychopath is an a-social aggressive, highly impulsive person who feels little or no guilt and is unable to form lasting bonds of affection with other human beings.' To this we could add an inability to learn from past experience, or to benefit from punishment.

Michael was the second son of a policeman. Like his brother, he was bright at school, but unlike him he showed no interest in going to university or embarking on a career. At 14, much to the embarrassment of his father he was convicted of setting fire to a parked vehicle while fooling around with a gang of older youths.

2 years later he was given 7 years' detention for grievous bodily harm on a sub-post mistress during a raid.

Despite an obvious attractiveness and likeability, Michael's nefarious career continued.

He is now serving a life sentence for the murder of a youth over a trivial argument. When questioned about his feelings on the incident, he shrugs his shoulders and laughs. He has no regrets.

Michael's mother is dead. His father blames him for his lack of promotion in the police force, while his brother, a practising lawyer, has washed his hands of him.

Michael is typical of the aggressive psychopath who causes such a headache to society. Many go to prison — a course of action which quite legitimately helps protect the public. Less nobly, it also exerts a measure of revenge while doing nothing to help rehabilitate the prisoner.

A psychopath more than any other patient will not want to change, and almost certainly will actively resist treatment. Hospitalisation may come about as a result of court action or because of a concurrent problem with alcohol, drugs or occasionally depression. Sometimes pressure from an individual, such as a wife or employer, may temporarily convince him of the error of his ways, but the psychopath's indifference to all but the gratification of of his own desires, means such interventions are usually doomed to failure. It is not unusual for staff to be initially impressed by the motivation and apparent enthusiasm for change in such a patient, only to discover that a further court case is pending and that he is hoping to impress those officials who must decide his fate. Not all pscyhopaths are aggressive. Some merely drift aimlessly along, appearing to need the strength of an institution around them, while at the same time exploiting its properties to the full. Some will be 'con' men of the highest calibre.

Janice, now in her early 30s, had a troubled childhood as the unwanted, illegitimate daughter of an alcoholic mother. A succession of hard drinking and unsympathetic men shared mother's life, but usually had nothing but contempt for Janice. Her early years were spent being dragged around public houses, being left unattended at home, or worse, being ill-treated by the adults around her.

Quickly she learned self-reliance, and by the time she was 7, she was a regular truant and accomplished thief. She frequently ran off in search of her father, who in her fantasy life was rich and kindly, but who in reality was unknown. She was demonstrably beyond her mother's control.

As Janice's need for care and attention became increasingly obvious, she was admitted to a short-term children's home. This heralded the start of her long association with institutions which has to date included spells in a variety of psychiatric hospitals and prisons.

At 15 she ran off with a 33-year-old alcoholic; travelling in stolen cars, they committed a total of 27 offences in six different counties before being apprehended for obtaining free board and lodgings in a well-appointed seaside hotel.

Apart from a 2-year period of comparative stability during which her own daughter was born, her life has been a continuing spiral of institutions, frauds and unfortunate sexual liaisons. She shows little sign of changing. Janice is a good example of an inadequate psychopath.

Not all psychopathically-inclined individuals go to prison, nor indeed are all prisoners psychopaths. A certain selfishness may be necessary to 'get on' and an oversolicitous conscience will be a great drawback in today's society. It seems undeniable that many prominent politicians or well-heeled businessmen owe their success to some extent to the personality characteristics described above.

Treatment

The treatment of psychopaths is absolutely fraught with problems, although some seem to improve gradually with age. Approaches, such as individual psychotherapy, which require the active co-operation of the patient are seldom attempted. The psychopath is likely to lack the commitment and forward planning to carry such approaches through. Long-term drug therapy is usually

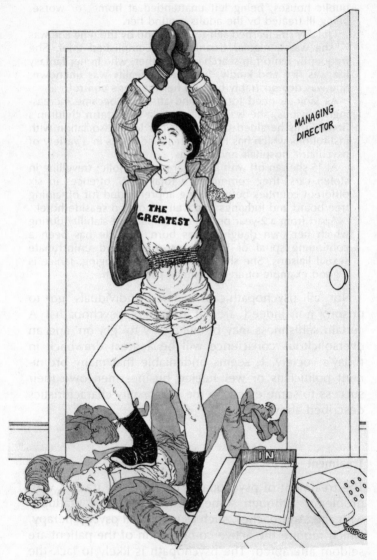

"I *am* the champion."

similarly unhelpful as the likelihood of abuse is consider-able. Superimposed depression, profound anxiety or withdrawal from alcohol may be treated by a carefully monitored, short-term drug regime.

Units specialising in the treatment of psychopaths are well-established, an early example being at Herstedvester in Copenhagen, as long ago as 1933. A physically secure unit is essential to prevent the patient 'opting out', but within the walls the atmosphere can be rigidly disci-plined or comparatively lax. The inmates will be given a degree of responsibility for their behaviour and for setting the ground rules. Psychopaths totally indifferent to the efforts of staff may sometimes conform to the rules set by their peers with whom they have so much more in common.

It must be appreciated, that because of past misdeeds and future possibilities the period spent in such units is likely to be lengthy.

NURSING THE PATIENT WITH A PERSONALITY DISORDER

By including all of the aforementioned under the blanket term 'personality disorder', the author could be accused of overgeneralising. Nevertheless, despite their wide diversity of needs, they do tend to present similar nursing problems often exacerbated by their *manipu-lative behaviour*. Some nurses may feel distinctly uncom-fortable dealing with these individuals. Unlike psychotic patients, vast areas of their functioning will be within normal limits. The very saneness of much of their conduct will render the rest of it frustratingly meaningless.

Nurses we can assume, experience much the same hopes, fears, aspirations and disappointments as the mythical 'man in the street'. They are liable to suffer hangovers, may detest getting up in the morning, can fall into debt or may be unlucky in love.

Most of them, most of the time, rise above such unpleasantness and struggle on with the work for which they are paid. It is not difficult to appreciate that they may be resentful if such work entails caring for the personality disordered patient. They may be more drunken, sleepier headed and deeper in debt than the nurse, but may seem oblivious to it all, as they flit from one sexual encounter to another.

The nurse must strive to recognise negative feelings in herself in order to put them consciously to one side as she cares for her patient. If she is moralistic or easily shocked she must take great care not to make it too obvious. Some patients may deliberately set out to antagonise the nurse so that should she finally react by becoming angry or rejecting, he can with some justification, claim, 'see, everyone's against me. Just what chance do I have?'.

On the other hand, some patients will consciously seek out one particular nurse. By deliberate flattery he may convince her that she alone can solve his problems and the nurse may become increasingly convinced that this is so. Little favours like tidying a locker or reheating a meal for a patient are simple enough procedures by themselves but may be subtle indications that the nurse is allowing a special relationship to develop. If the nurse finds she is becoming increasingly critical of her colleague's ability or if she finds herself becoming preoccupied with her contribution to one patient's care, to the possible detriment of others, she must call a halt. Discussion with other members of staff may reveal that they too felt 'special' or the only one able to understand this patient.

Patients who require hospitalisation because of manipulative behaviour in the community will not be helped if they can continue to employ it while in hospital. The nurse, therefore, is doing them a favour by confronting them with their actions.

As a result of her own prejudices and the foreboding of her more experienced colleagues, the nurse may be aware of her vulnerability to the tactics of patients with personality problems. Many nurses will have been conned in the past and will be unwilling to be caught out again. Yet to be unsympathetic is to deny patients their basic rights.

Of course nursing a patient with a personality problem is not just one long battle, but it does require some special skills. The nurse must be empathetic but firm; she must be flexible but capable of sticking rigidly to a treatment plan, and most of all she must be completely consistent.

Patients with personality problems require to have the rules firmly spelt out for them, with the opportunity to break them kept to a minimum.

In what has proved to be a difficult therapeutic area, most hope seems to lie in the therapeutic community approach, with its emphasis on personal responsibility and the group concensus. Learners nursing patients in this category should familiarise themselves with Chapter 8.

REFERENCE

McCord W, McCord J 1964 The psychopath. Van Nostrand, New Jersey

16

Anorexia nervosa

Miss Dukes suffered from anorexia nervosa.

In the month of July her periods stopped; she displayed a variety of psychological abnormalities and her appetite abated, although no physical cause could be isolated. She took to studying voluminously, poring over her books both day and night.

Morton, (her doctor) stated, 'I do not remember that I did ever in my practice, see one that was conversant with the living, so much wasted, like a skeleton only clad with skin, yet there was no fever, but on the contrary, a coldness of the whole body, — only her appetite was diminished, and her digestion uneasy . . .'

Miss Dukes was not a modern day victim of some 'slimmers' disease'. Perhaps the literary style is a giveaway. The doctor who treated Miss Dukes was writing in 1689!

Although difficult to classify, anorexia nervosa is usually described as a *psychosomatic disorder* characterised by a pursuit of thinness. Despite severe emaciation or debilitation, preoccupation and exaggerated fears about weight gain continue. Although isolated descriptions of the condition have been recorded for centuries, its prevalence seems to have rocketed in recent times.

The victim, classically a teenage girl, will usually present reluctantly for treatment, only after her life is threatened.

The appearance and physiological changes are listed in Table 16.1, and are consistent with starvation, whatever the cause.

Table 16.1 Characteristics of anorexia nervosa (physical)

Altered appearance
Emaciation (severe)
Poor peripheral circulation (extremities may be blue or purple)
Lanugo (i.e. fine downy hair on face and body)

Altered physiology
Amenorrhoea
Low basal metabolic rate
Hypotension
Bradycardia (possibly under *60* beats per minute)

Since many patients will initially come to the doctor's attention as a result of the weight loss or emaciation, they are likely to be seen by a medical consultant. However, some will first be seen by a gynaecologist for investigation of their amenorrhoea, and others may be referred directly to a psychiatrist.

Unspecific though the physical manifestations might be, (similar signs can be seen in inmates of concentration camps or victims of food shortages in third world countries), the psychological symptoms are typical only of the condition.

There is a marked preoccupation with food. Many anorectics are extremely knowledgeable about calorific values and the carbohydrate content of a wide variety of foodstuffs. Their interest in food may be partly indulged by taking over the family catering, by shopping for food or by planning elaborate menus. Many anorectics will express an interest in following a career in catering or dietetics. A morbid aversion to certain foods, typically carbohydrates, is likely to develop, and these will be

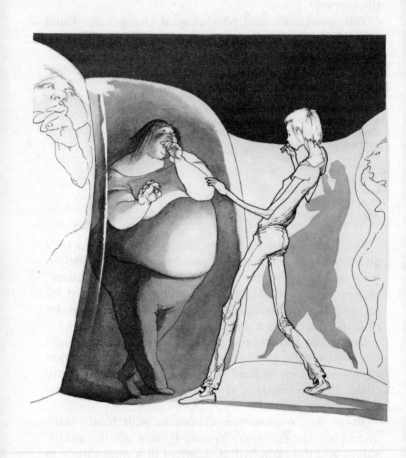

Mirror, mirror on the wall . . .

restricted, usually completely. The prospect of eating will herald feelings of apprehension and disgust, and if surrendered to, will leave the anorectic feeling profoundly guilty. Vomiting or excessive self-purging with laxatives may then occur. An interesting phenomenon, but one that is difficult for the nurse to understand, is the anorectic's apparent tendency to distort reality in relation to her body image. The nurse may be amazed to witness an adolescent who may be literally wasting away, viewing herself in the mirror and with great conviction, stating that she is fat. If asked, for instance, if she thinks she would be able to squeeze between two pieces of furniture without touching them, the anorectic may demonstrate just how distorted her body image is. She may have great difficulty in judging correctly, just how wide the space must be to allow her to pass through cleanly.

Despite her gross emaciation, she may carry out a testing routine of physical jerks, jogging in the shower, doing press ups in her bedroom and running round the block. This is calculated to burn off any excess carbohydrates she may have inadvertently ingested.

THE VICTIMS

Sufferers of anorexia nervosa are typically teenage girls, although they may present for the first time up until the age of 25. They are almost invariably of above average intelligence and are frequently very studious. Members of particular occupational groups such as models, dancers and actresses are especially at risk.

It is frequently said that anorexia nervosa is a disorder of the upper and middle classes and it is supposed to be much more common in privately run girls' schools than in their comprehensive counterparts. This class bias may be becoming less pronounced, and the fact that a small number of victims are male should not be overlooked.

CAUSATIVE THEORIES

The media

This is the 'slimmers' disease' theory, which rather simplistically assumes that the anorectic is a 'normal' dieter who has somehow gone too far.

Certainly the pressures on a young girl to be thin are very real.

Massive sums of money are spent on advertising one-calorie drinks, slimmer's breakfasts and weight watcher's soup and snacks. Each has the same implicit message: to be acceptable, you must be slim.

Products with no obvious links with weight control, such as washing powders, chocolate bars and even beer, are invariably advertised by slimline models. Lying on the sun-kissed beach, as depicted in the holiday brochures, likewise seems to be the prerogative only of the slim. Racks full of magazines cater for the weight-conscious, a countrywide network of self-help groups has been developed and matchstick-shaped models are idolised. In such an environment the girl who is not figure-conscious is the exception.

Attractive though it may be to make a scapegoat of the media and modern living, they cannot be deemed wholly responsible. It does not explain why only a tiny minority of youngsters develop symptoms when all are subjected to supposedly similar conditioning.

Intra-family conflicts

It is often noted that the interpersonal dynamics of a family that includes an anorectic are extremely complicated. Mother/daughter relationships are often especially tenuous, and the youngster often expresses a feeling of not being in charge of her own life. Paradoxically, should she start to lose weight dramatically, she may believe that here at last is one area over which she is genuinely in control. Fading away before the very eyes of her parents is a dramatic and anxiety-provoking action, which may be in part manipulative. Parents, driven to distraction, will try anything to get their daughter to eat and despite the inherent unpleasantness of her situation, she may feel it is worth the sacrifice in order to maintain this 'centre stage' position.

Family therapists, who prefer the concept of a sick family to that of a sick individual, would believe that the anorectic is merely the symptom of much wider malfunctioning. They would insist on treating the entire family, on the assumption that if the problems could be worked through, the need to produce a scapegoat in their daughter would disappear, and they could all function more healthily.

Flight from sexuality

An interesting theory is that anorexia nervosa represents an unconscious flight from sexuality or womanhood. In this it can be markedly successful.

Menstruation, that monthly reminder of her reproductive potential, ceases. The normal feminine curves disappear and rather unattractive hair appears on the face and body. Prospective suitors may be repelled. The onset of anorexia nervosa is said to be frequently precipitated by some event in the person's sexual life, whether during the sensitive teenage phase, or following an unsuccessful love affair or attempted seduction. The theory is that anorexia nervosa is an attempt to regain a childlike body in order to avoid adult sexuality and all its implications.

Consequently, the return of menstruation, an interest in heterosexual relationships, or marriage and child-bearing are considered healthy indications that the anorectic may be improving.

Male anorexia

Anorexia nervosa is very much rarer in men and consequently much less is known about it. A possible reason for its relative scarcity may be the fact that boys are known to be slightly older before they reach sexual maturity. This extra couple of years may mean that they are better equipped, intellectually and emotionally, to cope with their sexuality than are girls, who may be physically well developed while still very young.

Like their feminine counterparts, male anorectics may be fitness freaks, and spend a great deal of time weight-training, exercising or running.

BULIMIA

It has long been reported that many people who suffer from anorexia nervosa periodically go on *eating binges*. On such occasions, long episodes of fasting may suddenly be terminated by the uncontrolled intake of a large amount of foodstuffs, usually carbohydrates. This may take the form of a midnight raid on the family fridge. Such occurrences are usually accompanied by excruciating sensations of guilt and disgust and are likely to be followed by *self-induced vomiting* and laxative abuse.

In recent years more interest has been shown in this symptom and some dispute has arisen over whether anorexia and bulimia are two separate disorders that can affect the same individual at different times, or whether they are simply two phases of the one disorder. People subscribing to the latter view have suggested that the term **bulimarexia** should be used.

It has only recently been recognised that bulimia, with its attendant vomiting, can also occur in individuals of normal weight and it seems that this may have been overlooked in the past. The prevalence of bulimia in the population at large has not as yet been studied, but it could well be a favourite ploy of abnormal eaters to exert a degree of overall control.

Problems associated with the prolonged vomiting of bulimia are electrolyte imbalance/potassium deficiency which may cause muscle cramps, oedema, cardiac arrhythmias or myocardial infarction. The acidic content of the vomit predisposes to tooth and gum decay, which may require dental or medical intervention.

TREATMENT

Although anorexia nervosa is described in this chapter as being a psychosomatic disorder, the first step of treatment should be weight gain and restoration of nutrition. While this does not guarantee to cure the underlying problem, the cure cannot happen without it.

In practice a two-pronged attack is usually mounted on anorexia nervosa, with planned weight gain and psychotherapy being considered equally important. Although it is widely recognised that a grossly emaciated individual seems incapable of responding to psychotherapy, it may be unwise to withhold it completely until the target weight has been reached. To do so, may leave the patient with a body she disowns and a feeling that something awful has been done *to* her.

If an anorectic requires to be hospitalised, it is usual for her to be nursed in a single room. Here energy expenditure can be minimised, and the opportunity to hide food, vomit or otherwise deceive the staff is reduced. A target weight is agreed on and the relationship between therapist and patient is allowed to evolve.

Frequently a behaviour therapy type approach is used. This involves a system of rewards, as the patient makes the necessary weight gains. Initially, she may be denied all but the most basic amenities, and will be asked to draw up a hierarchy of privileges which she can subsequently earn. At first, moderate to large doses of chlorpromazine (largactil) may be prescribed, as this tends to control restlessness and stimulate the appetite.

As the weight increases, a more and more meaningful relationship should develop between the patient and her therapist, who, depending on his treatment philosophy, may at this stage wish to involve her entire family in family therapy, where they can explore their conflicts and areas of malfunctioning. Hopefully, this will allow the anorectic, on her eventual discharge, to go back to an environment which is much healthier than the one she left. However, since intra-family dynamics appear to play such an important part in the causation of anorexia nervosa, it is sometimes necessary for the recovered anorectic to find living accommodation elsewhere.

Gibson (1983) is very much against the behaviourist approach, which she considers degrading and dehumanising, and gives a valuable insight into why some anorectics may resist reaching their target weight.

'One of the anorectic's fears is that when she reaches a normal weight, everyone will assume all her problems has been solved. She needs to be constantly reassured that she will receive just as much care after gaining weight.'

Nevertheless, the behaviourist approach does seem successful in the short-term, although of course it is the long-term management that is most problematic. A good relationship between the former patient, her doctor and, when appropriate, the family is essential if it is to succeed.

A patient

Tanya was 14 years old and the younger daughter of a doctor and a physiotherapist who worked part-time at a local clinic. Her menarche had occurred just before her 13th birthday and her childhood development had been essentially normal. The daughter of intelligent parents, she excelled at schoolwork and was a very promising swimmer.

Following an apparently trivial piece of horseplay at the swimming pool, when some boy remarked about her figure, Tanya resolved to diet. She quickly reduced her carbo-hydrate intake until it was minimal.

Perhaps because mealtimes at home were irregular, perhaps because she developed great skill at pretending that she was eating when in fact she was not, or perhaps because her parents were too involved with their own problems to notice, Tanya was already quite emaciated before her plight was discovered.

Then, despite the rantings of her parents and the advice of their medical colleagues, her weight continued to plummet. Tanya was admitted, under pressure, to hospital, where she arrived clutching a vegetarian cook book and a keep fit manual. Amazingly, despite her skeleton-like appearance, she had just run three laps of the local rugby pitch.

She proved a difficult patient. Some of the nurses seemed sorry for her waif-like appearance and seemed to agree that her treatment regime was rather harsh. She bargained, pleaded and debated over every morsel, and was surpris-ingly successful at avoiding a bit of this and a bit of that. She was caught drinking excessively before being weighed, and found watering the ward plants with her supplementary high calorie drink. She argued so vehemently over her target weight that the therapist had to recheck its accuracy from another source.

Yet gradually, Tanya gained weight and following 10 weeks in hospital she reached her target. Eating now seemed to be slightly less stressful.

By the time she left hospital a month later Tanya had attended many sessions of family therapy. Sadly, these had been less than successful. Tanya's parents seemed to consider that she had been silly, that she was now cured and would take great care to see that it didn't happen again. They seemed unwilling or unable to explore the possibility of their own contribution and the home set-up has not substantially altered.

Tanya has made satisfactory weight gain but has failed to come to terms with her condition. Menstruation is still absent.

It seems likely that she will be back.

ANOREXIA NERVOSA AND THE NURSE

A major problem for some nurse learners will be the fact that many anorectics will come from an age group and family background similar to their own. They too may have counted calories and are even quite likely to have an anorectic among their friends or acquaintances. This can lead to overidentification with the patient, or conversely a lack of sympathy for someone who seems to be making a mountain out of the normal hassle of growing up. The need to develop empathic detachment (important in many psychiatric situations) is never more important.

Tanya's manipulative behaviour is typical of hospitalised anorectics, and the nurse must be very vigilant to detect surreptitious dumping of foodstuffs. Weighing should take place at pre-arranged intervals at the same time of day and on the same scales. The patient must wear the same nightdress (or preferably be nude) and care must be taken to ensure that she does not have heavy objects secreted about her person and that she has not been drinking massive amounts of water immediately prior to going on the scales.

This custodial aspect of nursing care can cause problems, in that it may recreate family situations with the nurse unwittingly playing the role of mother, or an envied sister.

In particular the need for a nurse to supervise mealtimes closely may colour subsequent nurse/patient relationships.

One answer may be to allocate a certain nurse to take charge of the eating aspects of treatment, allowing her to be fairly authoritarian. If she does not play a major part in the psychotherapeutic programme this will lessen the likelihood of tension overflowing from the table to the treatment session. An added advantage of this approach is that tensions and emotions shown towards the authoritarian nurse are likely to mirror closely those felt towards mother or an important figure at home. This can be ventilated and explored.

For the nurse thus involved, a certain degree of stoicism is required as she may unjustly become the recipient of her patient's anger. For the rest, consistency and caring is all important. The care plan should be carefully constructed and be made known to all in order to minimise the likelihood of staff being 'played off' one against the other, in an attempt to sabotage treatment.

Prognosis

Some anorectics appear to be cured, but the outcome in individual cases is difficult to estimate. Morgan & Russell (1975) studied 41 patients over a 4-year period and found good results in 39% and intermediate results in 27%, a poor result in 29% and death in 5%. Other studies have shown similar results, but caution is required in interpreting the figures. Of those reported to have done well or reasonably well, a significant number remained single, childless and living lives which many would regard as unnecessarily restricted or unfulfilled.

Summary

Anorexia nervosa is a condition which largely affects young females. Although recognised for several centuries it appears to have become more prevalent in modern times. Lately the symptom of gorging food uncontrollably, and subsequently vomiting it, has been increasingly investigated. This is termed bulimia and the question has been asked as to whether it is part of the same condition, or entirely separate.

Although the cause of anorexia nervosa is not fully understood and the treatment is lengthy, labour-intensive and unpredictable, a substantial number show at least moderate improvement. Others will die or do poorly.

In estimating how successful treatment has been, it is necessary to consider the quality of life, and to listen to the views expressed by the anorectic rather than rely entirely on the measurement of the body weight.

REFERENCES

Gibson E 1983 Body talk. Nursing Times 79:64
Morgan H G, Russell G F M 1975 article title Psychological Medicine 5: 353–371
Morton R 1689 Phthisiologica: or a treatise of consumptions. London.

PART | # FOUR

Wider issues

17

The perennial scandals — a possible explanation

Anyone who willingly works in a psychiatric hospital for a prolonged period of time is likely to become quite attached to the place. Authors of textbooks come into this category since the knowledge and experience that they hope to pass on will almost definitely have been accumulated gradually. Any sense of loyalty thrown up in the meantime should generally be applauded, although it can produce unexpected results.

Writers (having themselves contributed to it) will be aware of the vast amount of good work done in psychiatric hospitals and may feel disinclined to give publicity to unrepresentative examples of care that are less than exemplary. Consequently, chapters like this tend to remain unwritten. More sinisterly, the shared values and close knittedness of the staff can on occasion be problematic. When on the defensive, they can complicate investigations into complaints and make life difficult for anyone wishing to spotlight deficiences in care.

In the wake of periodic scandals which have disturbed and disappointed him, the author's personal experience convinces him that:

a. the overwhelming majority of psychiatric nurses, like other workers in psychiatric hospitals, are kindly, considerate individuals who consistently give of their best in sometimes very difficult circumstances

b. a tiny minority exists who may abuse their authority or deliver care of an unsatisfactory standard. Although rare, this occurs often enough to be alarming, and therefore, in the interest of patients cannot be ignored.

Over the last two decades a number of 'scandals' have erupted and the findings of several official enquiries are now available for general reading. Other enquiries have been completed in secret or have somehow been suppressed.

Problems have also arisen in hospitals caring for the mentally subnormal and seem remarkably similar to those occurring in psychiatric hospitals. Much of the following, therefore, is applicable to either setting.

Hospitals which over the years have been the subject of an official enquiry may now have acted on its advice. Sometimes, it has been said, that these hospitals are the unlucky ones, and close scrutiny of others might have unearthed similar deficiences of care. Consequently, we will not further stigmatise specific institutions which may already have suffered disproportionately to their crime. Instead we will consider common features unearthed by most enquiries and suggest possible causes. Beardshaw (1981) has already done this admirably, and her book, *Conscientious Objectors at Work*, is strongly recommended.

Specific complaints which crop up from time to time, include misappropriation of patients' food, money or luxuries, physical assaults on patients by staff and generally poor or insensitive standards of care.

Misappropriation of patients' property

In some ways this is the most clear cut offence. It is

indefensible but tends to be an individual thing for which the hospital milieu can only be partially blamed. Some people are dishonest and this unfortunately is also true of some nurses. The reason why it should be so is unclear, although Chapter 9 explains how some individuals develop a more punitive 'conscience' than others.

Nurses in charge of long-term patients may have almost unrestricted access to their money and property. Some patients will be completely unaware of their current financial status or even of the value of money. Obviously they are ripe for exploitation. Nurses who steal from patients are committing a serious offence which if detected would most likely result in dismissal, criminal charges and disciplinary action by the United Kingdom Central Council (UKCC).

On occasion, misappropriation of patients' property has been reported on a wider and semi-organised scale. Where pilfering is endemic, the possibility that the hospital set-up somehow lends itself to abuse must be considered.

Local policies may be woefully inept at safeguarding patients' property or providing a check on what they receive. In some hospitals a nurse in charge will draw the patients' money on his behalf and then be responsible for dispensing it. On-ward book-keeping may be rudimentary and even though a space for witnesses' signature is provided the process can easily be bypassed.

If 'Old John' needs money for tobacco it would seem inhuman to deny him until another member of staff was around to witness the transaction. They could sign for it later. If staff have no reason to doubt each other's integrity the need for rigid rule keeping may seem unnecessary, while more sinisterly, if more than one were dishonest, their criminal opportunity would be almost unlimited.

If the likelihood of being detected is demonstrably slight, it seems safe to assume that some individuals whose honesty is marginal will be tempted to steal. If theft is committed by a significant number of the staff it could almost become the norm and may again increase the chance of involving others. The development of a fool-proof method of accounting and an awareness of the possibility of misuse is essential, therefore, to protect patients and vulnerable staff.

Physical assault

The term assault covers everything from an ill-advised but playful 'cuff on the ear' to a fit teenager, to the systematic abuse of a helpless patient.

Assaulting patients can never be condoned, but it is useful to categorise incidents according to their possible cause.

It is recognised that caring for the mentally disordered can be extremely taxing. Wards can be understaffed, the shifts long and the patients unappreciative or obstreperous. In these circumstances, assaults may occur as a 'one off' happening. A member of staff, normally of good character, may momentarily lose self-control, or overreact in self-defence. When an offence has been proven the guilty party or his representative may strive to demonstrate that it falls into this category. If successful, he is likely to incur a less severe sentence and may even evoke some misguided sympathy.

At the other end of the scale, it is possible that an unscrupulous or sadistic individual could worm his way on to the staff. On psychogeriatric, long-term or mentally subnormal wards, the potential to exercise planned brutality is horrifying. It seems safe to suggest that only a tiny minority of nurses enter the profession in order to inflict injury on their patients. Nevertheless, the weeding out of such individuals, should they exist, must be a priority for everyone who may be in a position to spot them.

Most assaults are probably neither an understandable sequel to a specific event nor the calculated end product of a sick mind. Somewhere in between is a large grey area which accounts for the majority of these unacceptable incidents. Rather than being planned, brutality may evolve in conditions of apathy and poor supervision. When the atmosphere is generally uncaring and the short-term nursing aims unclear, a certain roughness may develop in some individuals. If allowed to go unchecked this can become the norm and a further drift into occasional overt violence may hardly be noticed.

Newcomers on the staff may be frightened to say anything, or worse still may accept these standards and perpetuate them in their own approach.

Treatment without consent may on occasion constitute a form of physical assault and is dealt with in Chapter 19.

Poor or inadequate standards of care

Very, very few nurses ever assault their patients. However the state of affairs described above as being the precursor of direct violence is itself unacceptable. In some ways, poor standards of care are as serious as theft and assault in that they are more common and less easy to legislate against.

By its very nature, nursing is an imprecise science and will remain so. We may abhor a colleague's tone of voice, which we perceive as derogatory, but what can we really do about it? Staff may degrade patients by talking down to then, calling them irreverent pet names or making them the butt of jokes or pranks of dubious taste.

In response to complaints they are likely to say that certain patients need 'jollying along' and that in fact, they enjoy being the centre of bawdy fun. They may even imply that it is the complainant who is insensitive to the patient's social needs. 'Things are different in Psychiatry.'

Ridiculous though this distortion of the facts may be, it can be very hard to disprove.

Other examples of insensitivity frequently reported by inquiring committees are: several patients being washed with the same flannel, dentures being kept out 'in case they go missing,' and a total lack of stimulation or diversion being provided on the wards.

Seclusion, the (usually illegal) locking of the patient in an empty or partially furnished room, is an extreme example of this.

Where the approach to *incontinence* is such that regular toileting does not take place, patients may suffer unnecessarily the degradation of wetting themselves. This will be made worse if they are not promptly changed or if they are castigated for their 'offence'. A lowering of the patient's self-respect and physical damage to the skin are likely accompaniments of such negative care.

Serious although each individual complaint may be, it is the tendency of 'scandals' to recur over time and with geographical variation that is most worrying. Allegations made at one hospital in the 1960s may be frighteningly similar to others made elsewhere much nearer to the present day.

Investigations into ill treatment in mental hospitals over the past two decades have on a number of occasions led to the suspension or prosecution of more than one person. This suggests that explanations concentrating on the individuals (e.g. momentary loss of control or innate 'sadism') are inadequate. What is it about mental hospitals that allows or apparently almost encourages breakdowns in basic care?

Several features seem to crop up regularly in the official inquiries.

Historically, mental hospitals tend to be self-contained, rather introverted units. In part this may have been planned since they were built (supposedly for the inmates benefit) far out in the country. In reality, this appears to have been an 'out of sight, out of mind policy,' aimed at protecting the sensitive Victorians from the harsh realities of mental disorder.

These institutions were large, and consequently required a substantial work force to run them. As a result whole communities emerged, largely geared to servicing the institution. It was, and remains, common for more than one member of the same family to work in such places, and for marriages to take place between various workers. At one time, promotion was mainly from within, with a tendency for staff to have to wait to 'fill dead men's shoes' before they could climb the ladder, almost strictly in turn. The terms 'nurse' and 'hospital' were foisted on such establishments and were not universally welcomed by those who worked in them.

Trade unions, like management, were sometimes dominated by certain families and frequently negotiators were personally well known to each other. Unions have tended to adopt the attitude that most episodes of malpractice can be laid firmly on the doorstep of management or the government, since they claim the root cause is poor working conditions caused by inadequate funding. Such conditions create the type of situation, they argue, where abuse can be anticipated and the bulk of the blame must lie, not with the individual abuser, but with the perpetuators of a system unwilling to pay a realistic price for the care of its weaker members. Not infrequently, trade unions have found themselves in the ambiguous position of having in their membership individuals accused of patient abuse and others who are making the accusations.

What effect does such insularity have on patient care? Familiarity, if not exactly breeding contempt, can foster attitudes of self-satisfaction or indifference. Unless there is a free flowing movement of ideas and staff, care can rapidly become routine and task-orientated. Such care which pays little heed to the individual nature of the patients' needs is more likely to encourage unacceptable standards.

It is however when malpractice is reported or suspected that the aforementioned properties of the institution and its staff can run most contrary to the interests of the patient.

Would-be complainants on the patients' behalf can be faced with a perplexing and apparently solid wall of indifference. Staff, loyal to the institutions whatever its shortcomings, are likely to cover up its deficiencies from the prying eyes of outsiders. They will be aware that they too are part of the set-up and that any adverse publicity will reflect badly on them.

Marriage or prolonged contact at work may foster a defensive solidarity between staff, union officials and management which can complicate investigations at the local level and leave complainants frustrated or even ostracised. Unions in their anxiety to protect their members from false accusations have on occasion left their other members, who saw fit to complain, feeling insufficiently supported and vulnerable.

The nurse's responsibility

It is not sufficient that the nurse herself delivers an excellent standard of care.

The fundamental responsibility of a nurse is to promote health, prevent illness, restore health and alleviate suffering.

> *The nurse takes appropriate action to safeguard the individual when his care is endangered by a co-worker or any other person.*
>
> International Code of Nursing Ethics, 1973

This, then, places a clear responsibility on the nurse to report inadequate care or nursing malpractice.

She may find the task neither pleasant nor easy.

Hospital management, whose overall responsibility nursing care is, will rightly expect that complaints should be made to them, and usually insist they are made as soon after the event as possible.

Nurse learners will find their tutors a valuable source of counselling and advice, as they are one step removed from the front line. Complaints should be made through the locally approved, formal channels, bearing in mind that some deviation may be required depending on who is being complained against. For instance, suggestions for improvement of on-ward care would normally be directed towards the nurse in charge but this would be pointless if she was seen as being the main offender.

If complaints through the official channels are frustrated, redress may be made to the Health Service Commissioner, Community Health Councils or the National Association for Mental Health (MIND).

Nurses who feel moved to make allegations about malpractice in hospitals cannot expect an easy ride but their decision as to whether or not to proceed must rest with their consciences.

Once again, the grey areas will be most difficult. Obvious physical abuse is unlikely to be tolerated by many nurses, but they may feel reluctant or powerless to act when what they witness is dubious rather than dangerous. If the standard of care is unsatisfactory in the eyes of the learner, but of such a nature that it cannot be proved to be illegal, she will hopefully try to improve matters by suggestion or example. If this fails, she has one remaining, overriding responsibility to her patients and herself.

She must, despite precedent or pressure, never allow her own standards to fall below what she knows to be acceptable. Nurses unhappy with the care in the ward on which they are placed, frequently find some solace and satisfaction in their insistence that their own efforts never waver from what they have been taught.

What hope for the future?

The above chapter is not meant to be alarmist. Scandals and their subsequent inquiries, although perennial, need not be inevitable. There is some indication that things may improve. Institutions are getting smaller. Their insular nature is gradually being eroded thanks, to a large extent, to the continual passing through of learners, some of whom are from other branches of nursing.

In the past it has often been student nurses who have highlighted inadequacies of care, but they have also more positive contributions to make. By reading, challenging and insisting on maintaining their standards they may gradually break down any close-knit tendency to outdated habits.

Promotions are now commonly filled competitively and although spending on the National Health Service is currently limited, care of the psychiatrically ill and mentally subnormal is considered to be a priority. The public and press, alive to the fact that things can go wrong, are alert and questioning.

Wards run on therapeutic community lines, where information flows freely and suggestions are welcomed wherever their source, make suppression of malpractices unlikely. Human rights is a topical subject.

Scandals in mental hospitals are abhorred by all who work in them. They damage public confidence in the system, threaten innocent workers and cause the old defensive barriers to be set up with renewed vigour. Yet like the Great Fire of London, they offer, when they occur, an opportunity to build again from scratch.

We must restate our emphasis on maintaining a sense of proportion. All mental hospitals are not punitive institutions, psychiatric nurses are by no means all sadists. Yet, too, we must avoid a sense of complacency. Where our charges are helpless and ripe for exploitation, an 'it couldn't happen here' attitude could literally prove fatal. We must be aware of the factors which may predispose to abuse and be ever alert for tell-tale signs of lowering standards.

We can never say that we have seen the last scandal, and a chapter such as this will long be required in psychiatric nursing textbooks. Perhaps the best we can hope for is that in future books it can be transferred from the 'current issues' to the 'historical' section!

SUGGESTED READING

Beardshaw V 1981 Conscientious objectors at work. Social Audit, London
Robb B 1967 Sans Everything, a case to answer. Nelson, London

The early days
Unilateral and bilateral ECT
Effect on memory
Consent to treatment

18

Controversial aspects of ECT

In its 'Memorandum on the use of ECT' (1977), the Royal College of Psychiatrists said: 'There is *substantial* and *incontrovertible* evidence that the ECT procedure is an effective treatment in severe depressive illnesses.'

Most psychiatrists probably agree with that statement and Electroconvulsive therapy (ECT) remains a common form of treatment in our psychiatric hospitals today. Yet no other procedure elicits so much emotion or attracts so much controversy as ECT — the planned administration of a therapeutic dose of electricity to the brain in order to produce an epileptic-type fit.

Perhaps many people erroneously believe that the only other time electricity is administered to human beings is during torture or judicial executions. If added to this, their mental image of epilepsy is one of a blood-stained individual, foaming at the mouth and thrashing uncontrollably on the pavement, it is easy to see why they view ECT with some distaste.

It is difficult to consider ECT unemotionally, but, when arguing for the treatment, the case is simple — it works!

For the type of depression described elsewhere as endogenous (see Ch. 12), particularly if the first episode occurs in middle age, ECT is said to be effective in over 80% of cases. Being relatively quick-acting it also shortens the duration of the depressive episode. Drugs, which at one time looked as if they might supersede ECT, can take upwards of a fortnight to work and this may be too long. Death by suicide could occur during the intervening period, while less dramatically, the patient is likely to suffer misery so abject as to be unjustifiable when a known cure exists.

The curative qualities of ECT are less in doubt than is its mode of operation. Its detractors make much of the rumours that it was supposedly discovered in an Italian slaughterhouse where it was used to stun pigs prior to cutting their throats. They are surprised that after 50 years, the use of ECT remains entirely empirical with nobody knowing how it works. When they add to this the fact that it was initially introduced as a result of the completely false hypothesis that schizophrenia and epilepsy are mutually exclusive, they believe that it is sufficiently lacking in scientific credibility to justify its ban.

Just why did ECT become so popular and why has it stood the test of time? ECT arrived on the therapeutic scene during a period when there was a dearth of available alternatives. Nevertheless, the gradual liberalisation of attitudes in general meant that purely custodial care was considered inadequate.

Enthusiasm had seemed briefly justified with the introduction of *deep insulin therapy* which however was to prove highly dangerous and largely ineffective. The schizophrenia/epilepsy argument, ridiculous though the passage of time may have rendered it, at least was based on something. For perhaps the first time ever, a real breakthrough seemed possible.

In practice, many, many patients received ECT, often on rather spurious grounds and surely it would have fallen into disrepute had not some of them got better!

In fact it transpired that it was those schizophrenics who tended to have superimposed depressive elements to their condition, who showed most improvement. Gradually, this has meant that the use of ECT has become almost confined to the treatment of depression.

It is not surprising that ECT became controversial. Originally, it was administered straight, (that is without the refinement of anaesthesia or muscle relaxants), making it both terrifying and unsafe. Side-effects included fractured limbs and crushed vertebrae as a result of the uncontrolled convulsions. Dental accidents and minor lacerations, while less serious, were commonplace.

Straight ECT was shown in the powerful film *One Flew Over the Cuckoo's Nest* and the result, although compelling viewing, did nothing to enhance confidence in the procedure.

Such portrayals are grossly misleading, while the motives for showing them must be questionable. After all, if we were making a film about the modern motor car, we would not use a pre-war model as an example!

The reality as we have seen is that a general anaesthetic is now invariably given as is a muscle relaxant. Patient discomfort is normally so minimal that it is common for them to awake during the recovery phase, asking when they will be having their treatment.

One of the reasons frequently put forward for giving ECT is the fact that it is considered safe. Although all patients nowadays undergo a strict physical examination before a course of treatment commences, there are few contra-indications. Nevertheless, patients who have dementia or any atherosclerotic condition or who are considered to be predisposed to them, are not normally given ECT. Similarly, this treatment is also withheld from patients with a history of recent myocardial infarction or cardiac arrhythmia.

The use of muscle relaxants means that pregnancy, old

age, hypertension and most orthopaedic problems no longer debar treatment, although each patient must be assessed for his suitability to undergo a general anaesthetic.

If we accept that the drugs often used as an alternative have themselves many potential side-effects and may on occasion be saved until they can be used in a successful suicide attempt, ECT's reputation for safety is further enhanced.

A common and apparently more justifiable criticism of ECT is the effect that it has on the *memory*. Reports of memory impairment, which are frequently made in both scientific studies and anecdotal accounts, require to be taken seriously.

Memories surrounding the day of treatment invariably seem to be lost, but a considerable number of people claim much longer-lasting and more serious impairments. A well-known author, who was later to kill himself, bitterly decried this aspect of ECT. He claimed that his memory was his 'capital' and that the treatment had put him out of business. It is frequently rumoured that members of professions, for instance doctors and lawyers, who are dependent on a good memory, are offered ECT much less frequently than unskilled personnel, and then usually as a last resort. This is difficult to prove as many doctors have in fact been treated with ECT. One (a practising psychiatrist, Anon, 1965) described his experiences thus:

> After the first treatment in both series, I felt a blunting of the acute sadness of the depression. Whereas before treatment I became fearful with very little provocation and felt intensely sad out of all proportion to the stimuli. After one single treatment I was no longer crushed by any chance sadness.

Of the memory impairment, he recalled meeting someone at a medical conference and remarking to his

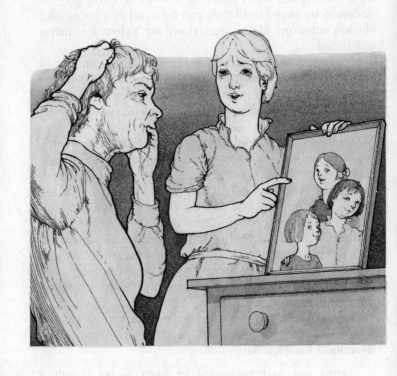

"Do YOU remember?"

colleague that the face seemed vaguely familiar. He was amused to be told by his companion that it should be, belonging as it did to the psychiatrist who had administered his ECT!

Unilateral ECT to the non-dominant hemisphere of the brain as described in Chapter 6 seems to have a definite decreasing effect on memory disturbance. Its therapeutic efficacy may be just as great as the traditional *bilateral* method and although further studies should be carried out, many psychiatrists believe that ample evidence exists to suggest that this should now be the method of choice. While transient memory loss following ECT may be so common as to be classed as normal, *confusion* is altogether more sinister. When it occurs it is often considered sufficient reason to discontinue the treatment.

Such complications are serious and raise the crucial question — does passing electricity through a healthy brain cause it any lasting damage? Critics of the treatment point out that neurologists go to great lengths to prevent their epileptic patients having fits because they believe it is bad for them. They see it as ironical, therefore, that psychiatrists deliberately set out to induce similar seizures in their charges.

Another significant complaint against ECT can be put down to the overexuberance with which it has been prescribed in the past. Due to a lack of alternatives, ECT may have been given frequently and, in retrospect, recklessly to large numbers of patients during the early days. We now know that many of these patients had little chance of responding but sadly the reputation of ECT suffered as a result. Its critics maintain that in the pre-phenothiazine era ECT was used too often in what seems to have been little more than an attempt to bludgeon retractive patients into some sort of compliance. Others believe it was used as a *punishment*.

If a patient was able to see or hear a colleague convulsing dramatically, or perhaps displaying signs of confusion or disorientation during the immediate recovery phase, he would be alarmed. If subsequently he was informed that unless he improved he too would require ECT, this constituted a threat. The use of such threats or the planned induction of fear has no place in modern psychiatry.

The giving and obtaining of *consent* prior to ECT has always been a thorny subject, yet it need not be so. The vast majority of patients enjoy informal status and are therefore subject to the same legal regulations as patients in a general hospital. Any procedure must be explained to them by the medical staff who must sign that they have done so. Informed, written consent must then be given before treatment can take place.

Irregularities are more likely when patients are being treated under a section of the Mental Health Act, that is the recommended patient. Yet the principles are similar. A recommended patient too must be asked to give his consent but of course may refuse thus placing the doctor in a difficult position. In the past when this happened doctors could and sometimes did give ECT solely on the basis of their professional judgement, but of course they left themselves wide open to charges of abuse.

The Mental Health Act 1983 has simplified matters and as such should be welcomed by doctors, patients and the champions of their rights. As we shall discover when we look more closely at this Act (Ch. 19) it is now mandatory for the doctor to ask for a second medical opinion before he can give ECT or other named treatments without the patient's consent. The doctor whose opinion is sought must in turn seek the views of two non-medical professionals (one of whom must be a *nurse*) who are both familar with the case. In good hospitals the need for consultation and the safeguarding of patients' rights have long been appreciated and practised informally. Now it has become obligatory.

Any incidence of patients being treated against their

will without the necessary legal requirements being fulfilled is indefensible. Moreover, it is probably illegal and the perpetrators should be sought out and prosecuted. Yet surely such happenings are not an inherent fault of ECT. The people, not the treatment, are to blame and ECT should not be condemned purely on such irregularities.

A more recent phenomenon has been the tendency for nurses to speak out against the use of ECT. In some cases individual nurses have gone as far as being sacked for refusing to participate in it. They would like to see the introduction of a *'conscience' clause* similar to that which already exists with abortions and which would give genuine objectors the right to abstain from taking part. There is no indication that this will be forthcoming.

Nurses who make a professional judgement and who are prepared to stand by it are to be applauded. It is perhaps the ability to do so that is in question. Are they influenced by emotion, or by politics? Granted that they cannot be called on actually to administer the treatment, can they morally refuse to give much needed nursing care beforehand, or during the recovery phase? If they succeeded with their 'conscience' clause would it open a flood gate? What else might someone object to in the future?

Conclusion

The controversy over ECT continues. Some see it as a degrading and unnecessary assault on the psychiatrically disordered. Others, who have already experienced its effects on their mood, plead to be given it again. In some hospitals patients refer to it simply as 'treatment' and think that unless they have been given ECT, they have not been treated.

Its detractors have asked how electricity passed through the brain can solve a patient's problems, whether they be with his wife or society. This is a red herring. Clearly it cannot rectify such problems. However when patients are carefully selected, medically examined and skilfully prepared, ECT can be a life-saver.

While acknowledging merits on both sides of the argument, the yawning gap between them at present seems unbridgeable.

One thing is certain — further studies, aimed at establishing its efficiency, refining the technique, diminishing the side-effects or finding more appropriate alternatives are continuing. They must be encouraged.

REFERENCES

Anon A Practising Psychiatrist 1965 The experience of electroconvulsive therapy. British Journal of Psychiatry III: 365

Royal College of Psychiatrists 1977 Memorandum on the use of ECT. British Journal of Psychiatry 131: 161

SUGGESTED READING

Mitchell R G 1983 Looking into the cuckoo's nest. Mental Health Forum, Nursing Mirror 156, (20): iii–v

Whyte L 1983 In our right senses? Mental Health Forum, Nursing Mirror 156 (20): vii–viii

19

Some legal aspects

Before considering the legal intricacies of caring for the psychiatrically disordered, two points must be unequivocally stated:

a. Legal acts and documents can probably only be fully understood by individuals qualified in the legal profession (the author has no such qualification).

b. Reading guidelines, potted versions or overviews of legal documents, including the Mental Health Acts, cannot compensate for failing to read the original version in its entirety.

THE NEED FOR MENTAL HEALTH LEGISLATION

Every society has its quota of eccentric individuals whose general mode of conduct is sufficiently outside the bounds of normality to be labelled 'mad', 'insane', 'abnormal', 'disturbed' or 'bizzare'. Thankfully, only a minority of such people require special legislation but for some, the need exists.

Some people cannot be allowed to remain in the

community at a particular moment in time. They may pose a danger to themselves, by neglect or self-injury, or may threaten the safety of others. They may be unaware of these dangers and may refuse to accept treatment. Channels must therefore exist to allow such people to be admitted, as a last resort, to hospital and to be detained against their will.

When this occurs, further legislation is required to ensure adequate human rights for those, thus stripped of their liberty. Laws which can broadly be seen as 'just' must be laid down regarding such eventualities as discharge procedure, the right of appeal, the prevention of exploitation (sexual, financial or other), consent to treatment and the general amenity of hospital facilities. Staff, too, must feel assured that if they act with professional competence and in good faith, they will be protected by the legal system.

The need for laws governing such matters is not seriously disputed and was embodied a long time ago, in for example, the now repealed Lunacy and Mental Treatment Acts of 1890 and 1930, and the Mental Deficiency Acts of 1913 and 1938. In the UK, the far-reaching acts of 1959 (England and Wales) and 1960 (Scotland) have recently been replaced by the *Mental Health Act 1983 (England and Wales)* and the *Mental Health (Scotland) Act 1984*. In Northern Ireland, similar but different legislation applies.

However, as none of these acts is exactly the same, and as in any case, they do not apply outwith the UK, it seems appropriate to concentrate on the broad principles they embrace. The alternative of peppering the chapter with a maze of figures relating to partially relevant sections and sub-sections is unlikely to be of much help. Readers requiring more detailed information must consult the appropriate acts, depending on the location of the hospital where they are employed.

Liberalisation of the Mental Health Acts

Perhaps the most dramatic and immediate effect of the 1959 and 1960 Acts was the overnight transfer to informal status of literally thousands of patients who, until then, had been legally detained. Some people still use the archaic terms 'voluntary' and 'certified' when referring to the legal status of patients, but these no longer exist. These acts introduced the less punitive sounding *'informal'* and *'detained'*, although the latter is sometimes substituted by 'compulsory' or 'recommended'.

Patients are legally detained only if they refuse informal admission and fall into the small category for whom hospital assessment or treatment is deemed essential. The proportion of patients legally detained has declined dramatically over the years since 1959, and it is believed that over 95% of psychiatric inpatients are now informal. In addition, those legally detained tend to regain their informal status after a much shorter period of time than was previously the case.

Compulsory admission to hospital

Various sections of the Acts allow for the admission and detention of patients. These include the short lasting *emergency admission*, an interim *28 days admission for assessment*, or the longer lasting, but carefully monitored, *'admission for treatment'* (sometimes colloquially called 'full' recommendation), and various court orders relating to individuals who are charged with or found guilty of a criminal offence.

In practice, application for the compulsory hospital admission is made by an approved social worker or the nearest relative as defined by the act, and is recommended by one, or more commonly, two doctors.

Emergency admission

This allows for the patient to be admitted briefly at short notice. The recommendation of only *one* doctor, usually the general practitioner, is required. This section of the Act should be used only in genuine emergencies where any delay would be undesirable.

> The family doctor was called to Margaret's house by her young son, Tony, who said she had smashed up her bedroom. Margaret, 34 years old, was interviewed in the middle of the upheaval while she was being forcibly restrained by two neighbours. She was tremulous, agitated and in a state close to panic. The damage to her property had occurred as she attempted to rid her bedroom of large rats which no-one else could see. Unable to do this and driven to the point of distraction, she had made a serious attempt to escape them by trying to leap from her window.
>
> Physically, she was dirty, undernourished and unkempt. There was no sign of food for herself or Tony. Margaret loudly refused the offer of informal admission, claiming that her GP, was 'one of them'. Nevertheless, her need for care and attention was obvious. Her doctor recommended that she be admitted compulsorily to hospital, where she was discovered to be suffering from alcohol withdrawal (DTs) and treatment was commenced.
>
> The emergency certificate is effective for only 72 hours, although in special circumstances the period of detention can be extended for up to another 28 days. However, as frequently happens, Margaret, by the time 72 hours had elapsed, was beginning to respond to treatment and appreciated the need for further hospitalisation. Consequently, no more legal action was required; she transfered to informal status and stayed to complete her treatment.

Admission for treatment

As it is not entirely satisfactory that one individual, however well-qualified or experienced, should have the power to strip another of a considerable part of his civil liberties, it is suggested that emergency certificates (with or without the 28 day extension) be used only in genuine emergencies. When the time factor is less vital, a recommendation that the patient be admitted either for assessment or treatment should be made by *two* doctors. Patients thus detained, can, subject to the considerable safeguards discussed below, be kept in hospital for a much longer period.

Psychiatry and the criminal offender

Psychiatrists and therefore psychiatric nurses will frequently be required to care for individuals who have been found guilty of a criminal offence or who have been charged and are awaiting trial.

Prior to the trial, the psychiatrist may have to assess the accused's mental capacity to plead, and/or withstand the rigours of the courtroom. After initial proceedings, the case may be held over until psychiatric or social work reports can be furnished. In some cases the accused may be found guilty but the psychiatrist may have submitted crucial evidence which could influence the type of sentence to be passed. Sentences ranging from community service, or probation on the condition that they agree to psychiatric treatment, to an indeterminate period of detention in maximum security may be considered appropriate in individual cases.

There appears to be a feeling among the lay public and perhaps others more closely connected with the legal system that the psychiatrist sets out to get guilty parties 'off the hook'. Particularly before the abolition of hanging, his role was extremely controversial. Largely on his say-so, it appeared, a convicted killer could be declared 'insane' thus denying the gallows a victim, and the vengeful public its pound of flesh. In England and Wales, the '*McNaughton Rules*', named after a deluded man who murdered Robert Peel's secretary in mistake for the then Prime Minister, are applied when deciding if a killer is insane. Roughly speaking, to get an insanity verdict, the accused would have to prove that he was not aware of what he was doing at the time of the offence, or if he was aware, he did not know that what he did was wrong. These rules are difficult to apply in practice, and are not used in Scotland.

Now that hanging is gone, some of the heat has been taken out of the situation, but controversy still remains. In recent years the verdicts in some of the most notorious murder trials have been determined by the so-called 'mad' or 'bad' argument. A section of the media appears to delight in selling a psychiatric verdict as being a soft option, and fuels the fears of the public who imagine that a dangerous killer may soon be returned, unpunished to the community. This ignores the stated opinion of several convicted murderers who claim to prefer a prison sentence (even a long one) with a known release date, to an indeterminate and possibly life-long stay in a 'special' hospital. As a necessary safeguard to the public, some individuals committed via the courts cannot be discharged as is usual, on the say-so of the consultant psychiatrist, but instead require the explicit authority of the appropriate *Secretary of State*.

It is the author's opinion (albeit a very personal one) that a lay jury is poorly equipped to pass judgement on a defendant's mental state. They cannot fail to be influenced by the popular myths of madness or to be puzzled by the occasional lack of overt symptoms in individuals on whose behalf a psychiatric explanation is being put forward. It is notoriously difficult to reconcile the apparently normal appearance of some people said to have severe personality disorders, with the lay concept of insanity, and seems disturbing that the jury can throw out the expert and even on occasions, unanimous evidence of a number of psychiatrists. Unarguably, there are many psychiatrically disturbed individuals at present housed inappropriately in our prisons.

Safeguarding patients from abuse

From time to time we here rumours of the apparent abuse of psychiatry in countries other than our own. It appears that some politically troublesome individuals have been incarcerated in a secure hospital on the pretext of insanity and are therefore denied a trial, a defence or even a known release date to which they can look forward. They can be 'treated' with large doses of tranquillising drugs, the prescription of which cannot be justified purely on medical grounds.

It is impossible to comment on the authenticity of these rumours, but equally, it cannot be denied that the potential for such malpractice exists. Due to the imprecise nature of much of psychiatry it can be almost impossible to prove that an individual is sane or otherwise. Perhaps the reader, like the author, is relieved that she is unlikely ever to be called upon seriously to convince others of the soundness of her mind. It could perhaps prove rather difficult! In the UK, there has always been, built into the Acts, considerable safeguards aimed at making abuses unlikely. The latest Acts have substanially increased these.

Apart from the emergency situation already discussed, two doctors must *independently* examine any patient before they can be legally detained. Moreover, one of them must be an approved psychiatrist, and normally they should not both be employed by the same hospital. In practice, it is usually the patient's own GP and the hospital psychiatrist who completes the necessary certificates and this seems to be ideal.

Apart from when court orders apply, periods of detention are clearly laid down, and further examinations by two doctors are again required before they can be extended. The Acts of 1983 and 1984 virtually halved the legal detention period which now stands at a maximum of 6 months in the first instance. This is renewable for a futher 6 months, and then at yearly intervals. The patient has clearly laid-down *channels of appeal* which he can use during each period of detention and which should be made known to him. Patients in hospital for an extended period will be automatically reviewed by an independent body at regular intervals, if they have not appealed themselves in the interim.

NURSE'S HOLDING POWER

For the first time, current Acts give certain trained nurses the right legally to detain an informal patient determined to discharge himself. They can only use this power, if it appears to them that the patient is suffering from mental disorder to such an extent that to leave would constitute a risk to his own or the public's health or safety. In addition, the doctor, (whose duty the ordering of such detention has always been in the past) must be unavailable.

This holding power, which in England and Wales covers a period of up to 6 hours, but only 2 in Scotland, has several implications:

a. It legally acknowledges the nurse as a competent professional, capable of making an informed decision. This is desirable from the nurse's point of view.

b. It replaces the unwritten, widely-held but untested belief that, even in the past, a nurse, acting in good faith and as a fellow citizen, could have detained an informal patient without fear of reprisal.

But,

c. In an era where the trend is correctly towards increasingly liberal attitudes towards the psychiatrically disordered, it vests in a whole new category of people (specified nurses) the power temporarily to deny the patient his liberty.

Any use of this power by a nurse must be carefully recorded with particular consideration being given to stating accurately the time at which it became effective. Efforts must immediately be made to contact the appropriate doctor, and on his arrival, the nurse's holding power will be invalidated.

CONSENT TO TREATMENT

The broad principle has always been that *informed consent* should be sought from patients before any treatment is carried out. Patients should sign the familiar form and the doctor must countersign that he has explained the procedure. This course of events has its parallel in general hospitals and, as a rule, works smoothly. However, there will always be some patients who refuse treatment that the doctor considers to be essential. These patients may be informal, or subject to legal detention.

Detractors of psychiatry and its carers, frequently and loudly decry the possibility of patients being treated against their will. The most recent legislation therefore, which goes some way towards clarifying what has always been a rather muddy area, should be welcomed.

Legally detained patients

While informal patients have a similar status to patients elsewhere and must normally give consent in writing, detained patients have had a different legal position for many years. Since the Mental Health Acts of 1959 and 1960 authorised the detention of patients in hospital for *treatment*, psychiatrists assumed that legal detention implied that such treatment could be given if it was in the patient's interests, whether or not they gave their consent.

This assumption was never challenged in court, although many pressure groups and individuals felt it dealt inadequately with the detained patient's rights of refusal.

Present legislation had to take into account the fact that compulsory treatment can be construed as a gross infringement of personal liberty, but on the other, that some patients, for the very reason that they are suffering from the condition which it is proposed should be treated, will be unable, or unwilling to consent to the treatment which is likely to be successful.

The new Acts allow for treatment which are not specifically mentioned, (presumably things like nursing care or OT) to be given **without consent**.

At the other extreme, treatments of special concern require the patient's informed **consent and** confirmatory **second opinions**, both medical and non-medical. This applies to all patients, whether legally detained or not, and covers such *irreversible* treatments as psychosurgery or the surgical implantation of hormones to reduce the male sex drive. Numerically, such situations arise very infrequently, in stark contrast to the intermediate position of treatments which require consent *or* a second opinion.

Treatment requiring consent or a second opinion

From time to time, certain treatments may be designated to this category which at present includes ECT and the continuous prescription of psychotrophic drugs for a period of more than 3 months.

If the patient has given his informed consent, treatment in this category may proceed. If the patient refuses his consent, but the doctor remains convinced of its necessity, an independent, **second medical opinion** must be sought.

This independent doctor, who must be approved for the purpose, must:

a. Examine the patient.

b. Consult two other people professionally concerned with the patient (one *must* be a nurse, and the other neither a nurse nor a doctor).

c. Certify in writing that the patient is incapable of understanding the nature, purpose or likely effect of the proposed treatment.

d. Indicate that the treatment should be given, since it is likely to alleviate or prevent deterioration of the patient's condition.

This guards against treatment such as ECT being given in the arbitrary fashion of the past, but also ensures that a patient will not be denied treatment just because his mental condition prevents him from giving his consent.

Once again, the professional accountability of the nurse is recognised. While in the past, psychiatrists could, and often did, choose to consult the nurse, such consultation is now obligatory. Nurses, however, must realise that doctors need not accept the proffered advice. They are required merely to seek it.

Patients need to be safeguarded against a great deal of potentialities and the influence of the Mental Health Acts infiltrates much of hospital life.

Other aspects of the Acts

A section of the Act makes it an offence for male nurses to have sexual intercourse with a female patient or to commit homosexual acts with a male patient. Obviously such a law is necessary and the penalty for infringing it is, rightly, severe. The exploitation of patients is absolutely reprehensible, although hopefully, the legal system is flexible enough to deal with the male nurse who may occasionally find himself caught up in circumstances altogether less clear cut.

Some female patients, who may be physically attractive, are sexually experienced, do all the running and seem quite capable of making their own decisions. An offence in such circumstances remains serious but could be construed as less detestable than one committed on a more helpless individual.

It is safest to steer clear of deep personal involvement with patients in this category and to avoid one-to-one encounters in circumstances which could be misconstrued or exploited.

A tiny number of patients may make malicious and completely unfounded complaints, incriminating a nurse whom they may either 'fancy' or abhor. The need to take all such complaints seriously, and to be seen to do so, means that the innocent nurse may be suspended and subjected to a harrowing experience.

Happily, such incidents are rare, but they are an occupational hazard when working with vulnerable members of society. The need for all nurses to be a member of a *professional organisation* or *trade union*, in order to safeguard their interests, must be emphasised.

Strangely enough, in this age of sexual equality, the possibility of a female nurse having sexual intercourse with a male patient does not appear to have been considered, and is therefore apparently legal. In practice, however, it seems likely that this would be construed as professional misconduct and that internal disciplinary proceedings would be initiated.

The scope of legislation dealing with the mentally disordered is far reaching. We have not considered how an individual may be appointed to handle a patient's affairs, or the laws regarding their sending or receiving of mail, including circumstances when it can be censored or withheld, and others when it most definitely can not.

Assault by staff on patients is a recurrent theme, and of course, patients, too, may assault fellow patients or staff. Can they be charged? Should they be sued?

Because of the all-encompassing nature of the Mental Health Acts, it is hardly surprising that they are wordy and difficult for the ordinary person to understand. They strive to protect the patient's rights, but at the same time, must protect the public from dangerous patients. They guard against unnecessary detention of a patient in hospital, but paradoxically, have made it possible for the nurse, in special cirucmstances, to prevent him leaving. They must cater for the weeding out of sadistic or undesirable members of staff, but at the same time, must offer protection to the very much greater number of caring psychiatric nurses.

Thankfully, in the UK, we have not reached the stage where we must be constantly looking over our shoulders for fear of infringing some piece of legislation, thus leaving ourselves open to civil action. Nevertheless, it is important that we have a working knowledge of the law as it currently stands.

I repeat my advice to readers that if interested, they should seek out and familiarise themselves with the Act that is appropriate to the country in which they are employed.

REFERENCES

Mental Health Act 1983 HMSO, London
Mental Health (Scotland) Act 1984 HMSO, London

The medical model
Introduction to alternative approaches
Psychoanalysts
Learning theory and the behaviourists
Conspirational, labelling and anti-psychiatry
models
Julie revisited

20

Alternative views

By now, any reader searching for the definitive description of psychiatry, psychiatric nursing or psychiatric disorder will have realised that she will not find it in this book. While the stated purpose of the author was to steer a middle course, some of the conflicting theories which abound must have become obvious. Ways of looking at theories of diseases and their treatment are sometimes called 'models' and there are many models used to explain mental disorders. Some are incompatible with others.

THE MEDICAL MODEL

It is common to be aware of this model only when it is being decried, yet despite being unfashionable it is still tacitly employed in many hospitals. Put simply, it states that psychiatric disorders are illnesses 'like any other' and should be handled in much the same way

In practice this means that the doctor is paramount. He requires a patient whom he can examine, to whom he can give a diagnosis and for whom he can prescribe treatment. He will feel more comfortable if he can announce a cause and confidently forecast a prognosis (the likely outcome). Rather unrealistically, patients, and perhaps even their doctor, believe that this outcome should invariably be a 'cure'. Sadly this is often impossible.

'For' the medical model

Individuals are ascribed the '*sick role*'. That is they are recognised as being ill and are expected to behave as such. People who are ill are, in return for seeking help and trying to get better, excused some of their responsibilities and absolved of blame.

This non-apportioning of blame is important; to be psychiatrically disturbed must be unpleasant, to be held responsible for that misfortune must be worse. A particularly distressing feature of some models is their tendency to apportion responsibility freely on others. It seems unnecessarily cruel to add to the already great burden of the parents of (for example) a schizophrenic teenager by accusing them of inadequate parenting, or labelling them 'schizophrenogenic' — a state which most probably does not exist. The sight of a family fumbling in the ideological dark, desparately trying to undo the imagined wrongs they have perpetuated is a sad one. Giving the patient the sick role negates the need for such arbitrary 'scapegoating'.

Another positive feature of the medical model is the fact that it is recognisable to prospective patients. Most people are accustomed to presenting themselves to doctors when things go wrong and are, to some degree, familiar with the bureaucratic rumblings of the health service. They may find it comforting in the event of psychological breakdown to be cared for within a framework they can recognise. To be told that they are ill may be a relief if they have been struggling to come to terms with a world where suddenly nothing seems to make sense.

Sometimes of course even 'experts' can be wrong.

The tale of a 'hypochondriac' being treated unsuccessfully by his therapist for years before dying of an undiagnosed tumour, is sadly too familiar. Doctors who use the medical model, on the other hand, will systematically look for all possible explanations of a condition, and will be alert to the possibility of a physical complaint being superimposed on the original psychiatric symptoms.

Lastly, of course, it is recognised that a large percentage of a GP's patients present with complaints, which are at least in part psychologically based. Similarly, it is a fact that most people with such complaints need never go further than their doctor's consulting room. This suggests that, for them, the medical model is acceptable and seems to work.

'Against' the medical model

Nevertheless it is widely considered that the medical model provides an inadequate solution for much of what we have come to call psychiatric illness.

Can a disease process always be demonstrated? Can the doctor explain schizophrenia? Can he cure alcoholism or accurately forecast the outcome of an affective crisis? Is it morally justifiable to ascribe sickness to an individual just because his ideals, beliefs or lifestyle may be substantially different from our own? Is the petty criminal any concern of the doctor and if so, why can't he 'make him better'?

The above examples highlight the fact that doctors cannot be all things to all people and are meant to question whether or not they should try. Certainly the medical model as applied to psychiatry is peppered with inconsistencies.

Some psychiatric hospitals operate 'black lists' of

patients whom they refuse to admit. Alcoholics can be discharged for exhibiting their main symptoms (i.e. they drink alcohol), although it would be unimaginable to throw out a cardiac patient who 'dared' to have chest pains. How many general patients would agree to pick potatoes or unblock lavatory drains as part of their treatment? Does a medical training really equip doctors to prescribe such 'therapies'?

Moreover, despite medical attention many patients show little improvement while some may even get worse. Has the cardinal rule been broken? Is the hospital in effect 'doing the sick harm'? Clearly, the medical model despite some advantages cannot satisfactorily contain or explain psychiatric disorder in its entirety. We may wonder why it continues to flourish.

The very fact that hospitals, doctors and nurses figure prominently in the bureaucratic process set up to manage the psychiatrically disturbed tends to perpetuate this model. Staff and patients may feel comfortable in it, and besides, by abandoning it completely, doctors are giving up their only legitimate claim to authority — superior *medical* knowledge and training.

By implying that many of the examples he has cited are ill, by including a classification of psychiatric illnesses and by concentrating on the efforts of doctors and nurses in influencing the process of change, the author has of course, in part, endorsed the medical model. The constraints of the syllabus and the expectations of the general nurse may partially justify this. After all, in a few short weeks it would be unnerving if not impossible to abandon entirely, the traditional roles.

Yet the overall theme of this book has been one of seeking, explaining and accepting a variety of approaches with the ultimate aim being the satisfaction of the patient's perceived needs. Amazingly, this could be considered controversial. The author believes that it is a matter of regret that psychiatrists from different 'schools' compete so dogmatically with each other, not noticing that they are thereby undermining psychiatry as a whole.

By seemingly demanding that any approach other than their own must be able to explain all life's nuances and be 100% successful before they will acknowledge its merits, they may be denying a lot of sufferers a lot of relief. After all, no one would claim that radiotherapy works for anything like all cancer victims, but it remains a well-used and, on occasion, dramatic treatment.

INTRODUCTION TO ALTERNATIVE APPROACHES

In discussing personality development, this book gives a lot of space to a psychoanalytical (mainly Freudian) viewpoint, but it acknowledges merit in many competing models. Often particular models come to be primarily associated with the most prominent people who espouse them and the remainder of this book will be used to introduce the nurse to outstanding individuals and their contribution to psychiatric understanding. The list is, of course, a personal one and cannot be considered exhaustive.

Other analysts

Many doctors began working with Freud and initially accepted his theories, only to reject or modify parts of them as their own ideas developed. Two early collaborators who were eventually to break with Freud to form schools of their own were Adler and Jung.

Alfred Adler (1870–1937) was to reject the concept of the Oedipal complex and greatly play down the importance of the unconscious. He believed that from an early age the individual strives for supremacy and much of his behaviour is determined by how he copes with his own perceived weakness. This he termed the '*lifestyle*'. Some individuals may choose a neurotic lifestyle in response to their weaknesses. This allows their 'illness' to excuse their lack of superiority, which in their fantasy can therefore remain unchallenged.

Carl Jung (1875–1951) formed his school of analytical psychology after disagreeing with the emphasis Freud put on infantile sexuality. He coined the terms 'introvert' and 'extrovert' and listed a variety of psychological 'types'. He remained a dedicated believer in the unconscious but stated that it could be subdivided into two, the *personal conscious* (with which we are familiar) and the *collective conscious*. Evidence of the collective conscious he felt could be found in the universal presence of certain myths and symbols in all cultures and religions. These he felt were somehow passed on from generation to generation and were indicative of a more primitive part of the personality.

As time passed Jung appeared to become less scientific and more mystical.

Learning theory and the behaviourists

The behavioural school is often considered to be diametrically opposed to the analytical one but it has been alluded to at various stages throughout the text. It is based on learning theory and put somewhat crudely, attests that all behaviour is learned. Behaviour considered maladaptive (e.g. symptoms of mental illness) could therefore be unlearned and replaced by more suitable conduct. The patient (if such he was) could then be pronounced 'cured'. The use of learning techniques in this way is called Behaviour Therapy and has been described in Chapter 7.

Ivan Pavolov (1846–1916), whose classical experiments with salivating dogs gained him a Nobel prize and a place in folk history, was a prominent pioneer of learning theory. Initially he noted that his dogs salivated when offered food. After a period during which they were given food to the accompaniment of the noise of a dinner gong, food was withheld. They continued to produce saliva however each time the gong was sounded. They associated the food with that particular noise and a conditioned reflex had been established. Such conditioning has been used to promote many theories as to how learning takes place, and may for instance explain seemingly irrational phobias.

Aversion therapy in which the individual comes to associate an unpleasant experience (vomiting) with the previously enjoyed ingestion of alcohol is an example of a conditioned reflex being used therapeutically.

J. B. Watson (1878–1958) an American psychologist applied Pavlov's findings to human learning in an extreme way. He rejected the existence of genetic heredity and claimed that a child was born with only a few simple reflexes. These became linked to new stimuli by conditioning and grew steadily more complex. Watson's belief in his theory was such that it allowed him to claim that given a dozen healthy infants and his own specified environment in which to bring them up, he could guarantee to produce at random any type of individual requested, whether it be a doctor, lawyer, artist, beggerman or thief!

Such claims seem exaggerated and risk bringing a lack of credibility to all learning theory.

B. F. Skinner (born 1904) has greatly influenced modern psychological thinking and has helped enhance the behaviourists' standing. His contribution has been in the field of operant conditioning, sometimes called learning by trial and error. Much of his work was done on experimental animals in so-called 'Skinner boxes'. By 'operating' on their environment, (as for instance by pressing a lever) the animal would receive a pellet of food as a reward.

This is called a reinforcer and means that the desired behaviour is likely to be repeated. Operant conditioning can rapidly induce animals to carry out a complicated variety of tricks, but more significantly can, as for instance in token economies, promote behavioural changes in individuals who may be considered mentally disordered. Behaviourist theories have a valuable contribution to make, both in the understanding and treatment of mental illness. It is unfortunate that they are often considered to be incompatible with other approaches since they can frequently bring about symptomatic relief. It seems unwarrantedly optimistic however to claim that something as complex as schizophrenia could be untangled and its victims 'taught' to become symptom-free.

Conspirational, labelling and anti-psychiatry models

Erving Goffman (1922–1983) is a Canadian sociologist whose name keeps appearing in the literature. He has been especially revealing in his consideration of total institutions and the effect on their inmates. Total institutions he described as being all encompassing and having inbuilt barriers to social intercourse with the outside world. These may be symbolised by the presence of high walls, locked doors or geographic inaccessibility. In 'normal' life people tend to sleep, play and work in different places, with different people under different authorities. There is often little formal communication between these different segments of their lives. In total institutions this is not so. All these activities take place under the same roof, in the company of the same 'batch' of companions and are timetabled in such a way as to meet the overall demands of the institution.

Some total institutions may be benign, such as homes for the blind, others like logging camps or army barracks may be largely work-orientated. Offshore oil rigs, for the duration of a spell on duty, form a topical example of a work-orientated total institution. Prisons and traditional psychiatric hospitals can be seen as being total institutions of a particularly unbending nature.

Goffman believed that the act of being in such an institution is stigmatising and itself counterproductive to psychological well-being. This labelling of deviants and their shipping off to institutions may directly result in more unusual behaviour which is then used as further 'evidence' to justify keeping them in the sick or 'insane' role. His emphasis on the adverse aspect of labelling, the stigmatisation of being an inmate and the propensity for institutions to perpetuate and exaggerate the behaviour which they are meant to contain is extremely valuable.

The author lives in relatively close proximity to a group of ex-psychiatric patients, who, after many years in hospital, have been successfully rehabilitated into a house in the community. He is impressed by their re-adjustment but similarly, he is aware of the pressure they are under to 'live down' their past. Eccentric, noisy or drunken behaviour on the part of the author or the rest of his neighbours, would if it occurred only infrequently, be allowed to pass almost unnoticed. On the other hand, if indulged in by the former patients, the self same conduct could be used as evidence that they are finally 'cracking up' again with calls to the hospital and demands that they be reincarcerated quickly being made on their behalf by their 'normal' neighbours. For an ex-patient, therefore, 'normality' is not enough. To undo their past, their adjustment must be extra special, and to some extent, they remain permanently on trial.

Goffman's work is invaluable in describing the sociology of life in an institution but his failure to acknowledge the existence of specific psychiatric illness (for instance, many of the inmates he described would be classed as schizophrenic by traditional psychiatrists) stretches his credibility rather far. He seemed to postulate that certain individuals were somehow arbitrarily designated as mental patients and were henceforth forced to live out their lives in total institutions. This has been called a conspirational model on the grounds that those in authority have conspired to pronounce a label of madness on those whose eccentricities offend.

Thomas Scheff. A sociologist working in America went as far as to state that labelling is the single most important cause of mental illness. A person whose deviancy cannot be easily categorised is described as being 'mad' or 'insane', a description which may stick with him for life. Once so labelled a self-fulfilling prophecy may be set in motion with the individual no longer acting responsibly even in his previously healthy spheres of influence, but instead, conforming to his designated role. Thus stigmatised, it can become extremely difficult to be taken seriously, as the experience of an intelligent lady briefly hospitalised following childbirth, illustrates. Ludicrous though it may appear, she was astounded to realise that her friends now placed much less weight on her philosophical or political arguments, although her personal difficulties were obviously entirely unrelated to any such matters.

Thomas Szasz. A Hungarian, domiciled in America, goes even further. Although himself a professor, a psychiatrist and a psychoanalyst, he is well known as a critic of psychiatry. He has frequently claimed that mental illness is a myth and even had to survive an attempt to sack him from his professorship, made on the grounds that he does not believe in psychiatry.

Szasz's extreme viewpoint states that whereas physical diagnosis, e.g. measles or bronchitis, involves the names of genuine diseases, psychiatric diagnosis does not. In psychiatry stigmatising labels are used to describe behaviour which offends us. Present day psychiatric treatment is merely a form of social interaction aimed at changing behaviour. A 'cure' is supposed to have occurred if this change in behaviour is in a direction of which we approve.

To Szasz there is no mental illness, only problems in living and psychiatrists, psychiatric nurses and psychiatric hospitals are therefore inappropriate. He believes that giving the patient, (a term of which he would disapprove) the sick role, is also inappropriate and a gross infringement of his rights. To say certain people are psychiatrically ill encourages apathy on both sides: the 'patient's' problems in living have been explained — he need no longer work at them, while society, by providing doctors and hospitals can absolve itself of further responsibility.

Compulsory psychiatric treatment he describes as torture, legal pleas of insanity or diminished responsibility, he fails to recognise. Somewhat incredibly, he believes that when a murder is committed, even by a person who would usually be considered insane, the perpetrator should be tried purely on the basis of his crime, with no consideration given to his so-called mental state. In fact, where the law allows, Szasz believes the murderer should be grateful if he is hung, thus preserving his dignity and avoiding for him, the stigma of mental illness!

While many people see nothing dignified in (for example) a schizophrenic hanging from the end of a rope, Szasz is influential and worthy of note. Perhaps his main contribution lies in his ability to shock the psychiatric establishment into continually reappraising its actions. Being labelled mentally ill *is* stigmatising, enforced treatment *can* be considered an assault and many patients *have* completely failed to benefit from the present system. But some would say Szasz goes too far.

Mrs W, described in Chapter 6, is typical of many people who develop depression in middle age and who make a spectacular recovery. Left alone, they would suffer unquantifiable misery and in many cases would kill themselves, (their right according to Szasz) but, if treated, they may well have many healthy, happy years ahead of them, possibly contributing substantially to their family or society. Yet they may refuse treatment.

The issues are moral and as such, have no easy answer. Szasz is a prominent member of the group known as *anti-psychiatrists* and his position as a psychiatrist, while at the same time denouncing all things psychiatric, is incongruous. Is he analogous to a policeman who does not believe in law and order, or a priest who is an atheist? If so, can he be surprised if not everyone takes him seriously?

Ronald (R. D.) Laing, who was born in Glasgow, is another controversial psychiatrist and psychoanalyst. The graffiti artist who wrote, 'Do not adjust your minds, there is a fault in reality,' sums up a major part of Laing's philosophy. He believes that schizophrenia can be a completely sane response to circumstances and that furthermore, it is a *'mind expanding trip'*.

Using detailed case histories of patients he had cared for, Laing decreed that parents of schizophrenics are unduly rigid in applying discipline in such things as toilet training. He claims that they restrict their children's freedom to grow up and limit their social or sexual opportunities. The 'double bind', where communications are ambiguous, is said to be common. An example of this would be the parent who unconsciously gives the message, 'I want you to disobey me.' It is obvious that any response could be wrong and in order to avoid punishment the young person may gradually divest his communication of meaning, since only by becoming incomprehensible can he avoid giving offence.

'Without exception,' Laing says, 'the experience and behaviour that get labelled schizophrenia is a special strategy that a person invents in order to live in an unlivable situation.' (his italics).

Traditional treatment could be construed as denying the schizophrenic his rich and positive experience and therefore would be seen as unjustified. Instead of damping down symptoms with tranquillising drugs the patient should be allowed to live through his psychosis under the auspices of a 'guru' or therapist who has preferably 'been there before'. This guided tour into madness and back, may lead to enlightenment, but would be considered by traditional psychiatrists to be fraught with the possibilities of suicide, homicide or irreversible psychosis.

Laing has produced no controlled studies to back up his theories, which although intriguing, must still be considered speculative. He has gained the reputation of being something of a cult figure, but has many detractors amongst traditional psychiatrists.

'Surely', they point out, 'a psychiatrist who doesn't believe in psychiatry, is the biggest double bind of all!'

JULIE REVISITED

What of Julie, whom we met at the beginning of the book and whose guided trip to the world of the psychiatric nurse this has been? A short modular experience and a short textbook, even in unison, cannot completely capture the flavour of psychiatric nursing. With her appetite whetted, Julie may decide that psychiatric nursing is truly for her, or like the majority of her colleagues she may return permanently to the general field. This is largely irrelevant. What is important is that she has developed some insight, empathy and an understanding of one simple fact. Whether intriguing, tantalising, frustrating or downright incomprehensible, psychiatric nursing is really all about people. That's why it is what it is.

SUGGESTED READING

Brown J A C 1961 Freud and the post-Freudians. Penguin, Harmondsworth

Burns R B 1980 Essential psychology. MTP Press, Lancaster

Goffman E 1961 Asylums: essays on the social situation of mental patients and other inmates. Penguin, Harmondsworth

Laing R D 1960 The divided self. Tavistock, London

Laing R D, Esterson A 1964 Sanity madness and the family. Tavistock, London

Seigler M, Osmond H 1974 Models of madness, Models of medicine. Macmillan, New York

Szasz T 1971 The manufacture of madness. Routledge, London

Wing J K 1978 Reasoning about madness. Oxford University Press, Oxford

Glossary

Acting out	the resolution of inner conflicts by anti-social or aggressive behaviour.
Affect	the mood.
Ageism	the assigning of unflattering stereotyped characteristics to, and subtle discrimination against, individuals, purely on the grounds that they are elderly.
Ambivalence	The co-existence of contradictory or mixed feelings, e.g. a wife who loves and hates her husband simultaneously.
Analyst	*see* psychoanalyst.
Behaviour therapy	a psychological treatment aimed at changing observable symptoms. It is based on the theory that all behaviour is learned and can therefore be unlearned.
Bilateral ECT	traditional method of electroconvulsive therapy (ECT) whereby the electrodes are applied to both temples.
Bulimia	eating disorder associated with anorexia nervosa. Involves sudden, excessive intake of food, usually followed by self-induced vomiting or laxative abuse.

Compulsion the intrusive and unwanted need to carry out a ritualistic piece of behaviour. The individual may realise this is unnecessary or illogical but will experience no peace of mind until he has done it.

Confabulation the filling of memory gaps with plausible fabrications. A common feature of amnesia induced by chronic alcohol abuse.

Crisis intervention action taken to minimise disruption following an actual or potential emergency, e.g. a visit to an 'at risk' alcoholic who has lost his job, or a group set up to explore the cause of a violent episode in a ward.

Custodial care a model of care which aims at merely containing the patient in order to protect either society or himself. Active treatment or psychological growth is neither sought nor encouraged.

Delusion a fixed, false belief which cannot be altered by reasoned argument. It is out of keeping with the individual's age, cultural background and level of education.

Desensitisation a method of behaviour therapy of proven value in the treatment of phobias. Involves gradually introducing the individual to his feared stimuli while he is in a state of relaxation.

Disorientation the state of being unaware of the hour or date (time), the identity of oneself or known other (person), or of one's whereabouts (place).

Dyskinesia (tardive) serious side-effect of some major tranquillisers. Involves oro-facial grimacing and involuntary movements of tongue, jaw and cheeks. May be irreversible.

Echolalia automatic repetition by an individual of words or phrases spoken to him.

Echopraxia   automatic and repetitive imitation of the movements of others.

Ego   the more mature layer of the unconscious mind which is most in touch with reality and which compromises between instinctual behaviour and the conscience.

Electroconvulsive therapy (ECT)   a common but controversial treatment for depression which involves the passage of a controlled amount of electricity through the brain.

Extrovert   a sociable, outgoing, impulsive and emotionally expressive personality.

Feelings of passivity   the belief that one is being influenced by others by means that are magical or telepathic.

Fixation   the arresting of the individual's psychological development at an early or immature level.

Flooding   an alternative method of treating phobias. Involves immediately confronting the individual with his most feared stimuli without any build up or preamble.

Fugue   a period of memory loss, during which the person wanders aimlessly and may even make a long journey. During this time, he may appear normal.

Group dynamics   the relationships, behaviours and interactions which customarily evolve when a number of people meet together with a common goal.

Group therapy   a psychological treatment in which a number of people meet together under the auspices of leader or conductor, to seek insight or gain symptom relief.

Hypochondriac   popular description of an individual who is preoccupied with ill health. His complaints may be either totally imagined or grossly exaggerated.

Hallucination a perception experienced in the absence of any stimulation to the sense organs. They may be visual, auditory, tactile, gustatory or olfactory.

Holding power (nurse's) the legal right of certain categories of nurse to detain informal patients in hospital for a short period of time until they can be seen by a doctor. The nurse must be convinced that to let the patient go would constitute a danger to himself or others.

Id the part of the unconscious mind concerned with primitive drives and instincts, e.g. sex, aggression.

Ideas of reference the belief by an individual that external events, e.g. television programmes, newspaper reports, have direct and special significance for him.

Illusion false perceptions due to the misinterpretation of a stimulus, e.g. a tap dripping at night may be mistaken for the noise of an intruder.

Institutionalisation a condition characterised by apathy, lack of initiative and submissiveness commonly seen in inmates of 'total' institutions, e.g. prisons, hospitals or work camps.

Introvert a withdrawn, shy, emotionally-reserved and self-absorbed personality.

Malingering the deliberate feigning of illness in order to gain reward or to avoid something unpleasant, e.g. work.

Mental defence mechanisms unconscious coping strategies used to protect the individual from anxiety.

Moral treatment a historically important change of emphasis in caring for the mentally ill in the 19th century, characterised by a kindly, more humane approach.

Neurosis immature attempt to adjust to stress. Abnormal emotional reaction in which

	the individual's talents and instincts may be inhibited, but during which he remains in touch with reality. The various types are classified by the symptoms displayed.
Obsession	fixed or recurring thought or impulse which is recognised by the individual as abnormal, but which cannot be willed away.
Oedipal complex	according to Freud, a crucial stage of personality development occurring around the age of 5 years. The child competes with the parent of the same sex for the exclusive affection of the other parent. When resolved unsatisfactorily, this situation may give rise to future psychological disorder.
Projective techniques	psychological method of treatment that allows individuals to express themselves indirectly, through painting, drama, pottery etc.
Psychoanalyst	highly trained therapist who facilitates awareness and change in individuals undergoing the prolonged psychological process of psychoanalysis. All psychoanalysts must themselves have been psychoanalysed.
Psychosis	a serious form of mental disorder involving a grave disorganisation of the personality. The perception of reality may be disturbed and hallucinations or delusions may occur.
Psychosurgery	any surgery to the brain, performed with the intention of relieving mental illness.
Psychotherapy	the so-called 'talking cure'. A psychological treatment requiring verbal communication and the establishment of trust and rapport between therapist and patient (client).

Psychotrophic medication   drugs which alter feelings, perceptions and behaviour without significantly influencing the conscious level.

Reality orientation   simple techniques aimed at diminishing episodes of confusion in the elderly by constantly and consistently reorientating them.

Reminiscence therapy   a form of treatment that aims to help orientate old people by encouraging them to recall their past.

Repression   the transfer of thoughts and memories from awareness to the unconscious.

Sadist   individual who obtains (? sexual) pleasure from inflicting physical or psychological cruelty on others.

Scapegoating   the apportioning of blame to an innocent party. In group therapy, the 'ganging up' of most members on an individual who becomes the butt of communal ill feelings.

Schizophrenogenic   a term used to describe an environment, home, family or most commonly a mother prone to producing schizophrenia in an individual. This theory is now largely discredited.

Sensitivity groups   groups where awareness can be enhanced and tensions worked through as a result of a free flow of comments and information. May be used to help minimise intra-staff conflict in a ward.

Sibling rivalry   jealousy or unhealthy competitiveness between the offspring of the same parents, i.e. brothers and sisters.

Stereotype movements   constant mechanical repetition of apparently meaningless actions.

Super-ego   part of unconscious mind which acts as an internal censor, the 'conscience'.

Therapeutic community a model of care based on a blurring of roles, free communications, frequent face-to-face meetings of patients and staff and a handing over to the patients of a substanial degree of responsibility for their own welfare.

Total institutions establishments such as prisons, psychiatric hospitals or work camps, which are self-contained and in which the inmates live a timetabled existance in 'batches' or groups.

Tranquillisers drugs which calm the individual down without making him fall asleep.

Transference the attributing by an individual of feelings and attitudes felt towards some significant person in his past to someone in a current interpersonal relationship. An important feature of psychotherapy.

Unconscious that part of the individual's psychological make up which is outwith his awareness and which cannot be controlled by will.

Unconscious motivation term used to describe the fact that individuals are influenced in what they do by wishes, drives and instincts of which they are unaware.

Unilateral ECT a method of electroconvulsive therapy in which both electrodes are applied to the same side of the head and the current is passed through the non-dominant hemisphere of the brain.

Waxy flexibility disturbance of muscle tone in individuals suffering from catatonic schizophrenia. This enables them to maintain their limbs in any position in which they are placed, however unusual or uncomfortable they may appear.

Index

309